Youth
SUICIDE

The School's
Role in Prevention
and Response

Phi Delta Kappa Educational Foundation
Bloomington, Indiana
U.S.A.

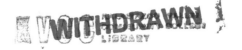

Cover design by
Victoria Voelker

Library of Congress Catalog Card Number 98-68592
ISBN 0-87367-812-5
Bloomington, Indiana U.S.A.

For
Dick, Eddie, David, John, and all youth
for whom life's passage has been too tortuous

Table of Contents

Introduction

Student suicides and attempts are among the most difficult experiences that educators encounter. In the past 35 years suicide among young people has increased at a greater rate than for any other age group: 300% for males and 230% for females (World Health Organization 1991). Studies indicate that at least half of all American adolescents have seriously considered suicide at some point before they graduate from high school. One in 10 students actually plans his or her own death, and virtually every minute a student attempts suicide — more than 500,000 attempts each year (Hicks 1990). About one in every 100 — or 5,000 annually — is completed. The disparity between completed suicides and attempted suicides may be a reflection of the ambivalence of suicidal youngsters. They can see no other way out of their problems but still have the desire to live.

Perhaps the most neglected segment of the youth population, gay youth, estimated at nearly three million of the nation's 29 million adolescents (Herdt 1989), represent a significant percentage of the adolescents who complete or attempt suicide.* Gay youth may be especially vulnerable to suicide because they experience greater social discrimination, depression, isolation, low self-esteem, and violence than do their heterosexual counterparts (Hunter 1990; Remafedi, Farrow, and Deisher 1991; Rofes 1983; Martin 1982). It has been estimated that from 5% to 30% of completed suicides are gay youth (Shaffer et al. 1995; Gibson 1989). Sources indicate that gay youth of both sexes are two to six times more likely to attempt suicide than nongay youth because of a lack of self-acceptance resulting from the internalization of a negative self-image and the lack of accurate information about

---

*Two comments about terminology are necessary. First, I use the term *gay* as inclusive of all sexual minorities: homosexual males, lesbians, bisexual and transsexual individuals. Second, current literature divides suicidal actions into "attempted" and "completed"; the term *commit* is not used with reference to suicide.

1

homosexuality during adolescence (Gibson 1989). A 1986 Department of Health and Human Services study, "Preventions and Interventions in Youth Suicide," leaves little doubt that public misunderstanding of homosexual youth has made a profound contribution to rising teen suicide rates (Gibson 1989).

No one knows for certain why young people take their own lives because, obviously, these youths are unavailable to tell us. Retrospective research indicates a variety of causes — and potential interventions. But there is a lack of consensus among suicide experts regarding the contributing factors to youth suicide. Different factors are emphasized by various experts according to their professional orientations. These factors include: psychiatric disorders (Berman and Jobes 1995; Shaffer et al. 1988), dysfunctional families (Brent et al. 1988; Capuzzi and Gross 1989), stressful life events (Garfinkle 1989), and drug and alcohol abuse (Brent et al. 1988; McKenry, Tishler, and Kelley 1983). Gay young people face the same risk factors for suicidal behavior that affect other youth: low self-esteem, family problems, breaking up with a lover, social isolation, school failure, and identity conflicts (Gibson 1989). However, these factors are exacerbated by other factors associated with homosexuality, such as social stigma.

A major factor in most teen suicides, regardless of sexual orientation and other issues, is loss of hope. Hopelessness, often reflected in depression, is a classic predictor of suicidal thoughts (called *ideation*) and, potentially, actions. Therefore, students need to learn how to recognize depression in themselves and their peers. And all adults in schools — teachers, counselors, coaches, administrators — also need to know the symptoms of depression. But recognition is not enough. They also need to know how to work with young people who are suffering from depression, how to communicate with them, and where and when to seek help from others.

Educators have important roles to play, which only they can accomplish, in both prevention of suicide and in the aftermath of a student suicide. First, they must become knowledgeable about the emotional and behavioral characteristics of students so that they can understand the pressures of normal adolescent development. This is a fundamental professional responsibility. They must be able to provide a consistent, mature perspective on the common emotional upheavals of adolescence. When a young person is experiencing emotional pain and despair, an informed and compassionate educator can offer encouragement and hope. That hope may be essential for the individual who, perhaps secretly, is wrestling with suicidal thoughts.

Second, because teachers spend many hours in direct contact with students, they can learn how to help students who are facing academic, family-related, interpersonal, or school-related problems. This is part of prevention, but it also is part of the needed response to a student suicide. In the aftermath of a suicide, teachers are in a good position to observe other students and to offer help to youth who are experiencing severe emotional reactions. Studies indicate that resilience to stressors, such as the death of a friend or family member, can be nurtured in youths who have even but one caring adult on whom they can depend (Werner 1989). Teachers, in particular, need to learn how to be that caring adult in a student's life.

A number of years ago the Phi Delta Kappa Issues Board identified adolescent suicide as one of several critical problems in education that needed attention. A result of that attention was the publication, *Responding to Adolescent Suicide*, released by the Phi Delta Kappa Educational Foundation in 1988. That monograph was developed by the Phi Delta Kappa Task Force on Adolescent Suicide and focused on the school's response to student death. In this book I have incorporated portions of that earlier work but with significantly greater emphasis on prevention. My hope is that if educators are more keenly aware of prevention strategies, then there will be less need for responses to student deaths.

As I stated at the outset, student suicides and attempts are among the most difficult experiences that educators face. The shock of a student's suicide, the sense of loss, and the grief permeate the school, the student's family, the families of the dead student's friends and classmates, and the community at large. Student suicide prevention is everyone's business.

While all students and educators are affected by the need to address suicide prevention, a student cohort that deserves particular attention is gay teens. The concerns of gay teens are not adequately addressed in the literature for teachers, school administrators, health care providers, and guidance counselors. Cultural taboos, fear of controversy, and a deeply rooted, pervasive homophobia have kept the education system in the United States silent on the subject of childhood and adolescent homosexuality (Uribe and Harbeck 1992). In fact, until recent years, the numerous studies done on adolescents and suicide failed even to mention gay youth (Gibson 1989; Proctor and Groze 1994). In the interest of justice and fairness, if for no other reason, the concerns of gay youth must be addressed.

My intention in writing this book is to create a resource that educators and others concerned about today's youth can use in developing efforts to prevent student suicide and, when such efforts fail, to respond in the aftermath of a student's death with concern, compassion, and competence.

Chapter One

ADOLESCENTS AT RISK

Why do young people, supposedly in the prime of life, take their own lives? If one asks this question of mental health professionals, the answer is: They have psychiatric problems (Shaffer et al. 1995; Berman and Jobes 1995). Yet research indicates that only about a third of adolescent suicide victims appear to satisfy clinical criteria for depression or other treatable mental illnesses (Centers for Disease Control 1996).

On the other hand, if one reads the accounts of adolescent suicides in newspapers, one gets the impression that *all* teenagers are at risk and that suicide strikes for no apparent reason.

Neither of these perceptions is accurate. True, a person with a serious psychiatric problem is at much greater risk of suicide than the average person. But many young people take their own lives who would not be diagnosed with a psychiatric disorder. Moreover, suicide is not limited to dysfunctional families or the economically disadvantaged. It can and does occur in strong and supportive families, and the affluent are not immune from risk (Colt 1991). In fact, many young people who kill themselves appear to be "happy-go-lucky" and free of problems. Only hindsight investigations show that these young people were struggling with enormous problems that they kept hidden.

Just as there is no single, general explanation for the 5,000 youth suicides that occur each year, there rarely is a single, simple explanation for any particular suicide. It may be just as true to say that a given adolescent chose suicide for a dozen reasons or a hundred — biological, sociological, and psychological factors that finally tightened like a knot around one place and time (Cantor 1987). The risk factors for suicide are that complex. And pinning down risk factors is exacerbated by the fact that most research is derived from suicide attempters, rather than from suicide completers. Risk factors for attempted and completed suicide may be different (Garland and Zigler 1993). But even given this complexity, it is possible to discern some common threads, and those bear noting.

AT-RISK INDICATORS

No single indicator is a sure sign of a teen at risk of suicide. But when a cluster of indicators can be checked, educators and parents should be alert to heightened risk.

- ☐ Poor school work; failing grades.
- ☐ Family instability; divorce.
- ☐ Death or illness of a loved one (including a pet).
- ☐ Lack of communication; inability or unwillingness to talk about feelings.
- ☐ Illness, chronic illness, or disability.
- ☐ Major disappointment; humiliation.
- ☐ Problems at home; lack of parent communication.
- ☐ Anger; feelings or expressions of a desire for revenge.
- ☐ Family history of suicide or suicide attempts.

Risk Factors

When students who have attempted suicide are asked, "Why?" they often respond: "It was a lot of things, some little and some big." More often than not, a combination of factors converge, and the individual reaches a point at which suicide seems to be the only way to escape. In some ways, therefore, the media-generated notion that all teens are at risk may not be far off the mark. Adolescence itself can be a complex of risks.

Teenagers often feel as though they are the only ones who ever experience bad things. This lack of a larger perspective allows them to believe there is no way out, that they are helpless, hapless, and hopeless (Elkind 1987; Wenz 1979). Adults often fail to understand the limited perspectives of adolescence. Adolescents may look like adults, but many teens are not able to think on an adult developmental level. They often are expected to act like adults but do not know how. They lack the life experiences that teach self-acceptance, patience, critical thinking, and an adult understanding that even the worst of conditions *can* change, that "now" is not "forever."

Another risk factor in general for adolescents is impulsivity. Adolescence is an impulsive age, and suicide often is an impulsive act. Young people with a history of impulsivity appear to be at greater risk than others. While impulsivity alone rarely leads to suicide, in conjunction with other life events it may increase self-destructive behaviors.

Depression, whether generalized or specific, makes one vulnerable to suicidal ideation, or the generation of suicidal thoughts. Adolescents show their depression differently than do adults, and so adolescent depression can be overlooked easily. The sadness and lethargy associated with adult depression may not be present. Instead, for example, a depressed youth may develop bodily complaints — headaches, muscle aches — or behave in ways that are referred to as "acting out," such as skipping classes, failing to do homework, or simply doing poorly in school. Acting out behaviors may be sufficient to get the student suspended from school. If a young person is depressed, either in reaction to a crisis or for reasons that are not apparent, he or she can be at risk of suicide. Depression combined with impulsivity increases the individual's vulnerability.

One often seen cause of depression is loss, which can be defined in a number of ways. For example, teens who experience the end of a relationship with a boyfriend or a girlfriend can see this event as a traumatic loss. Their sense of loss in such cases may be on par with more obvious types of loss, such as the death of a parent, sibling, or close friend or other relative. Divorce — the parents' end of a relationship — can engender feelings of extreme loss and disorientation in children and adolescents. And moving, whether an exacerbating factor related to a divorce or other traumatic event (such as a parent's loss of a job), can occasion feelings of loss, particularly if the teen moves away from long-term friends, has to enter a new school, or experiences other events that amplify the loss of familiar neighborhood surroundings.

This last point deserves particular attention, because it affects many young people, more than most educators realize. The United States is the most transient nation in the world. It is not uncommon to meet students who have changed schools four or five times. Moving, or having a friend move, is a stress factor — difficult for young children and even more difficult for adolescents. For some teens, the effect of frequent moves may be to diminish the teen's sense of belonging — anywhere. During adolescence young people form tight social circles of peers. Moving means leaving a familiar peer group and trying to find a new circle of friends, which often is difficult. Moving also means changing schools and getting used to new teachers and unfamiliar routines. It is easy to think that bright and gregarious students usually can handle such transitions well — indeed, they can — but they also may be even more anxious about fitting in, continuing to make good grades, and so on. Less confident students, whether academically slow or simply shy, may find such a transition overwhelming. Feelings of being unable to cope with moving can lead to isolation and feelings of worthlessness. Thus moving can be disorienting and stressful to the point of putting young people at risk of suicide.

Any disappointment can become a risk factor that, combined with other risk factors, can lead to suicidal ideation. Many teens do not confront disappointment well; and any setback, from a poor grade to not making the cheerleading squad, can be blown out of proportion. Inability to cope realistically with disappointment makes some teens emotionally vulnerable. At the same time, such teens may be unable to reach out to parents, who often

Depression Alert

Educators and parents who suspect that a teen may be depressed should look for one or more of the following indicators.

- ☐ Declining school performance coupled with expressions of apathy or helplessness.
- ☐ Sudden loss of interest in pursuits (sports, hobbies) that previously were a source of pleasure.
- ☐ Abrupt change in behavior, such as sudden reckless driving or an attempt to run away from home.
- ☐ Marked change in sleeping or eating habits, such as excessive sleepiness or loss of appetite.
- ☐ Lack of communication or a sense of alienation from friends or family.
- ☐ Withdrawal from social contacts; desire to spend excessive amounts of time alone.
- ☐ Impulsiveness or uncharacteristically erratic behavior.

Indicators suggested in Mary Giffin, "Cries for Help," *Guideposts* (July 1980): 32-35.

are preoccupied with career requirements in an era when few parents have the luxury of staying home. Adolescents are left with more free time and less supervision than in past eras, and this combination of factors can prove to be lethal for some teens.

Free time, lack of supervision, and, in some cases, a ready source of money also can lead to substance abuse. While the use of illegal drugs, overuse of prescription drugs, and alcohol abuse do not cause teen suicide, they are nonetheless powerful indicators that trouble exists. For a depressed young person, the temporary "high" of drugs or alcohol is a dysfunctional coping strategy that provides a brief "escape," only to be followed by a decline into depression. Use of drugs or alcohol, and any change in such use, should raise a red flag for the parents, teachers, and friends of the teen user. The purposeful overdose of drugs, legal or illegal, as a method of suicide is seen more often in females than in males. But any habitual substance abuse can be a factor because such use reduces inhibitions that might otherwise keep the teen from completing a self-destructive act.

Two additional factors bear mention. Young people with a chronic illness or a handicapping condition also should be considered at risk. Many adolescents are obsessed with personal appearance; anything that sets them apart from their peers is a source of great concern. Even temporary conditions that affect personal appearance — such as acne or delayed physical development — can create stress because adolescents do not view these conditions as temporary. Chronic, long-term illness or a physical handicap can put a youngster at risk even if the condition is relatively "invisible." A young person with diabetes or hemophilia, for example, may still feel "deformed" in some sense and may feel like a misfit among other youth (Elkind 1987).

Finally, adolescents who have suffered physical, sexual, or emotional abuse must be considered to be at risk. Abuse destroys a young person's sense of self-esteem and often leaves him or her with profound feelings of guilt. This can be doubly true for gay youth who have no support group and may not be well-accepted by peers or family. Belonging to a social group and maintaining self-esteem within that group are basic human needs (Maslow 1970).

Gay Youth at Risk

I single out gay males and lesbians because the adolescent suicide rate for these young people is far out of proportion compared to the general teen population suicide rate. It has been estimated that suicides by gay youth constitute from 5% (Shaffer et al. 1995) to 30% of completed youth suicides annually, and gay youth are two to three times more likely to attempt suicide than other young people (Gibson 1989). These statistics are not surprising considering the verbal and physical abuse gay youth often suffer from their peers, families, church, and society solely on the basis of their sexual orientation (Anderson 1994; Gibson, 1989; Hershberger and D'Augelli 1995; Procter and Groze 1994; Schneider et al. 1989; and Uribe and Harbeck 1992).

The suicide risk factors for gay youth are similar to those for nongay youth, but they are magnified because of the hostile environment many gay youth must endure. Gay teens, whether they conceal their sexual orientation or are open about it, tend to experience greater social discrimination, depression, isolation, low self-esteem, and violence than their nongay peers — all of which sharply increases feelings of desperation that can put them at risk for suicide (Proctor and Groze 1994).

Schools often are unsafe environments, places where openly gay or suspected gay youth are reviled and abused; and far too often educators turn a blind eye to the problem. But if schools are unsafe, the same may be doubly true at home. Many gay youth experience a strong negative response from their parents, for whom the discovery that their child is a homosexual feels like death (Johnson 1996). Consequently, the young person's sense of isolation may be doubled. And many gay youth become runaways or "throwaways," further adding to the already high risk for suicide.

One need not draw a complex portrait of extreme risk to realize that the most vulnerable adolescent is one who is depressed, impulsive, gay, and has experienced several negative life events. However, any young person attempting to cope with severe emotional problems, alone or in ineffective ways, needs assistance. Whenever teachers become aware of a young person who feels isolated, who has no way to find a peer group, who is facing a series of traumatic events or a major, one-time crisis, they should be alert for emotional fallout and be informed, able, and willing to offer help. As I will suggest later in this book, that help can take many forms. It can be as simple as putting the hotline number for a suicide crisis center into the hands of the student or his or her family or friends.

Cluster Suicides

Before concluding this chapter on risks, I should say a few words about cluster suicides. Adolescent suicides that occur in clusters in the same geographic area and over a short period of time are both puzzling and frightening. A romantic fascination with death is normal for adolescents, but currently there is no clear explanation for why the suicide of one teenager may trigger others to do the same. What is known is that young people who take their lives in these situations do not always share the characteristics of the at-risk suicidal adolescent identified by research.

Although there is no satisfactory explanation as to why cluster suicides occur, one factor often associated with them is the accidental death of a student known in the community. There also is evidence that when the media report suicides and give a full description of the methods used, the same methods have sometimes been replicated by the cluster suicide victims. The problem is complicated when reports by local media are picked up by national syndicates and networks. For example, in 1987 when four teenagers took their lives with carbon monoxide poisoning in New Jersey, similar incidents quickly followed in Illinois, Nebraska, and Virginia. No one knows how many attempts may have been made during the same time.

Several communities have formulated guidelines that may be helpful in curtailing cluster suicides, though it is not known how effective they are. Cluster suicides seem to end as mysteriously as they begin, and no one is certain which actions, if any, make a difference. But certain activities help to pull people together in a community and serve as a calming influence over what could be a panic situation. Following is a list of suggestions from communities that have dealt with cluster suicides:

1. After consultation with the family, school officials should contact the local media and seek their cooperation in not reporting the deaths, except in the obituaries. If the media consider this to be a restriction of press freedom and do not agree, request that

they make their reports as brief, accurate, and neutral as possible and, further, that they report the measures the school and the community are taking to cope with the event. School officials also can issue press releases to assist the media.

2. School personnel should collect the names of the deceased students' peer group and see how many students are mutually acquainted. All students known to two or more of the deceased should be considered as a high-risk group.

3. School officials and local mental health personnel should create a protocol for suicide/depression evaluation or obtain a depression evaluation instrument, such as the Beck Depression Inventory. Then officials should obtain parent permissions to assess all students in the high-risk group. The protocol or evaluation instrument should ensure that all interviewers ask for the same information. Community mental health professionals should be asked to help; many will volunteer to assist in this kind of crisis. However, it is best to use licensed practitioners — school or mental health — and to ensure that they are covered by malpractice insurance.

4. After the evaluations are conducted and the high-risk group has been further delineated, school and mental health officials should determine the types of support that are available to this group from families, friends, and agencies.

5. For those students at greatest risk, officials should enlist at least four adults who are willing to serve as monitors — perhaps two at school and two in the community. Two or three times each week, each of these monitors should spend at least five or ten minutes with each at-risk student, in person or on the telephone, and ask specific questions in a direct manner. Youth tend to be open and give honest answers when confronted by someone who really cares about their welfare (Hicks 1990). Specific questions include: How are you? Are you getting all your homework done? Are you seeing friends? Are you eating regularly? Do you have any sleeping problems? What are you going to do this weekend? The answers to such basic questions can alert the monitor if the student is having trouble with basic day-to-day functioning.

Should that happen, then the monitor can contact parents, teachers, and others who can step in and better support the student until the crisis passes.

6. High-risk students also can be asked to join discussion groups for six to eight weeks. These need not be specifically "grief" groups. Rather, it can be most useful to provide a forum where all issues can be discussed — academic, social, and personal.

7. In addition to working with the media and students directly, it is imperative for school officials to conduct regular information sessions for parents. Parents are likely to be anxious, and their anxiety can be projected to their children. Some parents will want to blame school officials for the deaths. Such feelings can be dispelled by keeping open the channels of communication between school and home. It will be reassuring to parents to know precisely what efforts the school is making to deal with the situation.

Risk, by its very nature, is difficult to define. No single factor puts a student at risk of suicide, but every suicidal ideation arises from an individual complex of factors. In this chapter I have tried to delineate some of the factors that seem to be most prominent in cases of attempted or completed adolescent suicide. Sometimes, as in the case of cluster suicides, ideation appears to arise impulsively, making the suicide of one young person a factor in the suicide of others. In spite of the complexity of risk and risk assessment, knowing that such risks exist and being able to spot them are important information for educators, who often are in the best position to help students avoid those risks.

Chapter Two

OBSTACLES TO SCHOOL-BASED SUICIDE PREVENTION

In Chapter One I identified some of the risk factors that school officials need to be able to recognize and, in the case of cluster suicides, what they can do directly as preventive and responsive measures. One purpose for writing this book is to help educators develop school-based suicide prevention programs. However, developing school-based suicide prevention often means overcoming a number of obstacles. Therefore, before I take up the development of a school-based suicide prevention program in Chapter Three, I will use a few pages to describe those obstacles, assuming the validity of the cliché that forewarned is forearmed.

Death and suicide are difficult issues. They raise up cultural stigmas, particularly when the death is that of a young person. And suicide, often viewed culturally as a sin or a dishonorable act, makes that death an even more uncomfortable event, something with which most people would rather not deal.

Avoidance and denial regarding youth suicide can limit appropriate responses. Parents may refuse to discuss potential risk factors; they may not see the risk factors as being related to the potential for suicide. And they may be unwilling to talk about suicidal behaviors even though such behaviors can be more lethal than sex, drugs, or alcohol. Parental reluctance often translates into a similar reluctance on the part of school officials, who may fear a parent backlash.

When homosexuality as a suicide risk factor enters the picture, the walls go up even more strongly. The taboos and stigma associated with homosexuality and teen suicide can be sufficient to threaten the security of school officials. Indeed, some school administrators "opt out" by claiming that teen suicide is a mental health issue that is beyond the scope of schools (Cochran and Turner 1986). In fact, this is not the case. Only about a third of adolescent suicide victims appear to satisfy clinical criteria for depression or other treatable mental illnesses (Centers for Disease Control 1996).

Nonetheless, suicide prevention may be the last item on the school officials' agenda, because homosexuality — and adolescent sexuality in general — is such a sensitive issue. In many cases, schools do little or nothing in terms of outreach to gay youth because homosexuality is still viewed as a taboo subject. Many school officials will readily admit that they are unaware of problems facing gay students; but given the tenor of our time, such an admission must be viewed as willful ignorance.

The stigma of homosexuality also inhibits the inclusion of gay issues in the curriculum, prevents the formation of gay youth support groups in schools, and sweeps the problems of young people who are struggling with questions of sexual orientation and identity under the schoolhouse rug. For example, a recent survey of school districts in Ohio found no district tackling gay youth issues in any significant way (Schleis and Hone-McMahan 1998). Some sources believe there is a bottom-line paranoia among school administrators who wonder, "How many angry parents would I have on my head if I got too out-front on gay issues?" (Aarons 1995). Such administrators are likely to believe that it is "safer" to bury their heads in the sand and pretend that gay issues do not exist.

Safer for them, perhaps; but it is hardly safe for young people, especially gay adolescents. The reality is that gay youth represent a significant number of youth who attempt or complete suicide (Herdt 1989).

Invincibility and the Vicissitudes of Youth

One of the problems inherent in dealing with youth suicide is the attitude that young people are invincible. Teenagers tend to think of themselves in this way, which often accounts for reckless behaviors. But adults, too, often see young people as indestructible and view their problems as minor, something to be chalked up to the vicissitudes of youth.

Unfortunately, the same absolutism that makes most young people think they are invincible also follows in the negative. When things go wrong or problems arise, the problems are likely to be viewed as insurmountable. Adolescents can jump rather quickly across the fine line between hopeful and hopeless. And it is a sense of hopelessness that often leads to suicidal ideation.

Adolescence is the point at which young people need to develop critical thinking and problem-solving skills. And it is the developmental point when most teens do develop such skills — but not all. Critical thinking and problem-solving skills are vital for adolescents to weigh and evaluate the stressful events that may temporarily affect their lives (Elkind 1987). They are the skills that allow teens to see such events as temporary, rather than permanent and therefore hopeless.

Unfortunately, this developmental need may not be recognized and the so-called invincibility of youth can blind friends, families, and teachers to suicidal behaviors. A case in point: When a 17-year-old Ohio youth gave away his prized leather jacket to a friend, his family believed that it was simply an act of generosity. When this same youth placed his usually unkempt room in perfect order, his parents believed he had simply decided to do much-needed cleaning. And then this boy killed himself.

In reality, giving away prized possessions is one of the warning signs of impending youth suicide. The same is true for acts that can be construed as making final arrangements, such as suddenly straightening an ordinarily messy room (Giffin 1980). Actions that appear slightly unusual but, on the whole, rather ordinary can — and should — be red flags for those who understand the risks and symptoms associated with youth suicide.

Deciding whether a youth's behavior is significant in terms of suicide risk sometimes is a difficult call, because behavior changes can be indicative of a variety of adolescent stresses. Often a common denominator in youth suicide is that the young people usually tell someone, most often a friend, of their self-destructive intentions (Berman and Jobes 1995; Ross 1985). But, again, too often such revelations are put down to the individual "being dramatic" or exaggerating his or her misfortunes.

This is another obstacle to prevention under the guise of the vicissitudes of youth. Parents and educators may slough off suicide as "unthinkable." But students do think the unthinkable. And, in fact, all suicidal comments and threats by young people should be taken seriously. Such utterances should trigger prevention program efforts.

The more difficult situation is the silent threat, and these are the cases where a prevention program can be even more valuable. Teachers and administrators need to be informed about suicidal ideation and behaviors. They need to be able to distinguish between ordinary, non-suicidal behaviors and behaviors that may indicate that a student is at risk for suicide. Another case in point: An honor student began simply sitting in the classroom without participating. Instead, he gazed out the window, signed his test papers without attempting the problems, and failed to complete his assignments. Teachers and administrators' only "treatment" for this youngster was detention, which did not help. The student's school experience continued to deteriorate, and the student killed himself.

What the educators and parents in this case failed to realize was that the student was severely depressed. A student, more often than not, will not say, "I'm depressed." Instead, he or she will act out, either by being disruptive in school or by withdrawing mentally and emotionally, which was how the student in this case behaved. Perhaps if the school had developed a suicide prevention program, this student's behavior might have been noticed for what it was: a red flag that the student was at risk for suicide.

Depression is a classic risk factor; and no matter how resilient young people can be, they are not immune from depression. As one writer described it:

> When emotional burnout and depression seep over a soul, nothing in life seems worthwhile. Nothing. Not family, not friends, not work, nothing. All seems pointless. Then it's almost as if troubled people stand before a window in life, one through which they must pass to begin life anew, refreshed. For some, the window is large and the passage not too difficult. For others, the window is narrow, the passage torturous. (Range 1986)

The Stigma of Homosexuality

Gay youth disproportionately attempt and complete suicide. Therefore, it will behoove educators to pay particular attention to issues surrounding adolescent homosexuality, because such issues form a nexus of obstacles to youth suicide prevention.

Homosexuality and suicide share similar societal burdens of religious and social stigma. Various factions see both as "sins" or associate both homosexuality and suicide with mental illness. As a result of these views, openly gay youth, young people who "act gay," and adolescents who are struggling with sexual orientation and identity questions often are reviled and subjected to harassment on a day-to-day basis that most adults would find unbearable (Anderson 1994; Gibson 1989; Proctor and Groze 1994; and Uribe and Harbeck 1992).

In many cases, in order to avoid harassment and hostility, many gay youth in schools attempt to be anonymous and silent — even when help, such as a gay youth support group, is close at hand. For example, a 14-year-old Ohio youth, prior to his suicide, confided to his friend that no one at school must learn that he was gay because he would be beaten up, that every day he feared for his life. This same youth did not attend the local gay support group, which met within a few blocks of his school, because he feared the other kids at school would find out (Mallet 1997).

Gay youth learn, often painfully, that in order to avoid harassment and abuse, secrecy is critical in a society that insistently preaches the evils of homosexuality (Hammelman 1993). This secrecy itself is another obstacle to suicide prevention. Because of such secrecy, gay youth are not always known to school personnel and caregivers involved in suicide prevention efforts. Invisible to service providers, gay young people often experience greater social discrimination, depression, isolation, low self-esteem, and violence than do their nongay peers (Proctor and Groze 1994). Such invisibility leaves them to face the risks unaided.

The stigma of homosexuality creates several obstacles that complicate, or intensify, the perils of adolescence, such as attitudes of invincibility. Not least among these obstacles is lack of training for those educators who are ready and willing to look beyond homophobia. Indeed, most educators desire to be part of the solution, rather than part of the problem, for gay youth. But many are hampered by lack of training about gay issues because such issues are still too often regarded as taboo subjects in schools. For these individuals, ignorance, not indifference, is the obstacle to acting effectively (Ross 1987).

Lack of Knowledge and Curriculum Compatibility

Not only is educator knowledge of homosexuality issues inadequate, but so is knowledge of suicide in general. This is another obstacle to be overcome in developing an effective suicide prevention effort. Some studies indicate that the training most teachers receive is cursory and ineffective and suggest that suicide is a topic that should be included in teacher preservice training. Preservice training would allow more time to be spent on how to recognize suicidal behavior, how to react to a student's confidence, and how to make referrals (Sandoval, London, and Rey 1994).

Coupled with such training must be work on values, because the value orientations (perceptions, feelings, attitudes, and priorities) of principals, teachers, and counselors are critically important variables that directly influence school-based suicide prevention and response programs (Bennett 1996).

Too often, administrators and school boards also question whether suicide prevention efforts are compatible with curriculum goals and whether schools have the resources to implement such programs. They may not view suicide prevention — or homosexuality awareness — as a priority when considered along with academic subjects and meeting state education requirements.

An Ohio health teacher for eight years recently told me that homosexuality has never been a topic in his class, except during lessons about AIDS. He said, "I don't see it as one of the major issues. As a teacher, you pick and choose what is the most relevant to most of the kids." A former board of education member related that "schools are taking too much of the social, moral teaching away from the parents. Schools should concentrate more on academics than. . . social teaching" (Schleis and Hone-McMahan 1998). These self-limiting attitudes shunt student safety to the sideline — and make schools unsafe places for many students.

The Mental Health Obstacle

Because sources differ on the most effective approach to youth suicide prevention, the various arguments can become obstacles in themselves. A good example is the debate between a mental health perspective and a stress reaction perspective. Although they are not mutually exclusive, these perspectives are distinct.

The mental health perspective is that there is a link between suicide and the youth's mental health, which may be impaired by depression, antisocial attitudes, or substance abuse. Thus mental "illness" is the key factor in the individual's suicidal action. The mental health perspective often is viewed as most appropriate simply because the greater amount of research in youth suicide has been accomplished by psychiatrists studying youths admitted for suicide attempts (Proctor and Groze 1994).

In contrast, the stress reaction perspective is that suicide may be considered by any youth as an option when faced with extreme stress. I noted earlier that this perspective often is conveyed by the media and, in fact, seems to be more prevalent in schools.

Both of these views can limit effective prevention: the former because it depends on a judgment of mental illness, the latter because it says that all students are potentially at risk, rather than looking more critically at specific risk factors. But in reality, most suicides that are attempted or completed occur because of a complex of factors. Some form of mental illness may be at work and stress may be its cause, but either-or propositions do little more than clutter the landscape.

The mental health perspective can be a particularly thorny obstacle because it can allow schools to see suicide prevention efforts as beyond their scope. If suicidal behavior is viewed as mental illness, then schools may — in their view, rightly — claim ignorance, schools not being clinical settings (Bernhardt 1984). Moreover, parents also may fail to see their children as being at risk for suicide unless the youngsters show definite signs of mental illness. Thus denial is available: "Not my kid." And prevention efforts will be blunted.

The fact is that whether youth suicide is seen as a mental health issue or not, it is distinctly a health issue. However, in spite of the attention given to youth suicide since the 1970s, it is not regarded as a major public health problem. Statistically, youth suicide is considered a rare event (Grazman 1991), even though it is one of the top killers of our youth (Wolfle 1997). In 1994, for example, suicide was the third leading cause of adolescent death, exceeded only by accidents and homicides (National Center for Health Statistics 1996).

Political and Financial Obstacles

Finally, political considerations and limited finances often become obstacles to the development of an effective suicide prevention program.

There often are financial limitations that keep schools from implementing school-based suicide prevention programs. In addition, there is a political disincentive for schools to implement these programs. Public schools are political entities that depend on public funding; consequently, programs as controversial as suicide prevention may be difficult to fund. Thus schools opt for passive or reactive approaches.

A few words must be said about why suicide prevention programs can be viewed as controversial. One aspect that I already have discussed is the link between gay youth and suicide. Sexuality always raises the specter of political problems. But an additional factor that may argue for silence on suicide prevention is the parental fear that open discussion may introduce the idea of suicide to teenagers who have not thought of it previously. This argument follows the logic of not teaching about sexual matters for fear of "planting" ideas in teens' heads, an argument that holds little water in our media-soaked environment.

Schools also often feel pressured by so many professional development issues that time and resources for training teachers in yet another area may be difficult to obtain. Thus, because they involve a relatively small number of students, gay issues and teen suicide may be given lower priority as topics for staff training. But there is a larger picture to consider: Dealing with isolation and depression among students — key concerns in dealing with gay youth and teens at risk of suicide — also can help other students who simply need help to feel better about themselves. This is an area that should not be left to the schools alone. As I suggested previously, teacher training institutions might provide leadership in developing awareness and competence for both preservice and inservice professionals.

Schools also may run scared on the basis of legal liability concerns, particularly in the event of a student death (Jennings 1989). However, some mental health professionals stress that schools should be more worried about the potential liability involved in *not* offering any type of suicide prevention program. The Ninth Circuit Court of Appeals decision in *Kelson* v. *The*

City of Springfield, 1985, demonstrated that a school can be held liable in connection with a student's suicide if the school does not have an adequate suicide prevention program (Colorado State Department of Education 1990).

MYTHS ABOUT TEEN SUICIDE

MYTH: Teenagers who talk about suicide don't complete suicide.

FACT: Of any 10 teenagers who kill themselves, eight have given definite warnings of their suicidal intentions.

MYTH: The suicide rate among teenagers is so low that there is no need to be very concerned with it.

FACT: Many "accidental" deaths among teenagers would be ruled suicide in adults who can communicate distress more easily.

MYTH: Teenage depression is quite rare; but when it does exist, it is very similar to adult depression.

FACT: Teenagers become depressed relatively frequently, but their depression is quite different from that of adults. Their depression often is "masked" in other behaviors; typically the teenager will engage in "acting out" behaviors.

MYTH: Teenagers, like adults, have well thought-out plans if they are seriously suicidal.

FACT: Teenagers can be very impulsive and may attempt suicide after a seemingly minor incident. Also, the most commonly chosen suicide methods of teenagers lend themselves to impulsivity.

MYTH: Teen suicide happens without warning.

FACT: Studies reveal that suicidal teenagers give many clues and warnings regarding their suicidal intentions.

MYTH: Suicidal teenagers are fully intent on dying.

FACT: Most suicidal teenagers are undecided about living or dying but gamble with death, leaving it to others to save them. Almost no one completes suicide without letting others know how they are feeling.

MYTH: Improvement following a suicidal crisis means that the suicidal risk is over.

FACT: Most suicides occur within about three months following the beginning of improvement, when the individual has the energy to put his or her morbid thoughts and feelings into action.

MYTH: All suicidal teenagers are mentally ill, and suicide is always the act of a psychotic person.

FACT: Studies of hundreds of genuine suicide notes indicate that although the suicidal teenager is extremely unhappy, he or she is not necessarily mentally ill.

MYTH: Suicide occurs much more often among the rich or, conversely, among the poor.

FACT: Suicide is neither a rich person's disease nor a poor person's curse. Suicide is represented proportionately among all levels of society.

Adapted from "Facts and Myths of Teenage Suicide," Suicide Prevention Center, Inc., Dayton, Ohio. Used by permission.

Chapter Three

DEVELOPING A SCHOOL-BASED SUICIDE PREVENTION PROGRAM

In the previous chapter I discussed some of the obstacles that educators face in developing youth suicide prevention programs. That collection of obstacles was by no means comprehensive. Indeed, any effort to establish a school-based suicide prevention program is likely to face stiff odds for the reasons I stated but also because we do not know with certainty what to do to keep young people from killing themselves. It is discouraging to realize that suicide prevention strategies have been implemented in a number of areas since the 1970s and yet the youth suicide rate continues to rise.

One factor we do know is that the suicide rate increase correlates with the increase in alcohol and drug use among the young, greater availability of firearms, changes in the nuclear family and society (Berman and Jobes 1995), and increased stress experienced by the young (Garfinkle 1989). Clearly the issues are mingled, and only a multifaceted effort to keep young people safe in the broadest possible sense will avail.

At the same time, predictable stages of youth suicide and the presence of common risk factors lead many experts to believe that suicide among young people, though enormously complicated, often can be predicted (Shneidman 1985). It is this predictability of suicidal behavior that gives hope for prevention.

Predictability of Youth Suicide

Young people on the road to suicide often go through predictable stages and exhibit commonly recognized signs of their suicidal intentions. For example, direct verbal statements, often dismissed or overlooked, are probably the most obvious signs. A young person might say, "I don't want to live anymore," "I'm going to kill myself," "I wish I were dead" — utterances that adults and other teens may put down simply to adolescent angst and overdramatizing.

An Ohio youth told his friends that he was going to end his own life by the water. They dismissed his words as "fantasy." Later, this youth took his life under a bridge over a river. This same youth had made several significant indirect statements. For example, when his grandfather wanted to buy him a fishing license for the next year, the youth said, "I won't be needing a fishing license any more." He often said to his friends, "I feel as useless as a stone being kicked along the street." On the morning of his suicide, he refused his weekly school lunch allowance from his mother, saying, "I won't be needing money this week."

Another predictor of potential youth suicide is unexplained behavioral changes. Take the case of an honor student who suddenly seemed unable to concentrate in class. He stopped doing homework and began to receive failing grades in all of his classes. Like other suicidal youth, who often express sadness or melancholy in their artwork or writing, two days prior to his suicide this 17-year-old wrote the following poem.

I was through a woods the other day
And I saw tiny flowers sitting among the brush,
and I wondered as to their cause, for it seemed so small,
they have colors that are so perfect
that I wondered how such colors could come about.
But is it needed for everything to be explained,
Rather than to marvel at its beauty?
It is the cause of a tiny flower to shed light, how so ever small,
Upon a world of opulent darkness.

Yet I am no bigger than the flower, and I wonder,
Could it not be the meaning of life?
And I came to think that flower was indeed a wiser thing
(to be so selfless as not to fight)
selfless and rendering when being picked.
Beauty that is above all beauty,
And silence that is above all understanding,
And in my view, an understanding that is above all inherent to
    man.
It quietly stands unwanting to move, yet on and giving to all who
    pass by.

Given these kinds of verbal and behavioral indicators — along with the risk factors I discussed in Chapter One — most schools that do anything in terms of suicide prevention opt to develop school-based programs that focus on one or both of two levels of activity:

1. Teaching staff and others to recognize suicide indicators and to help at-risk students obtain appropriate mental health care.
2. Helping staff and others to address risks directly to reduce the potential for youth suicide.

The first level of activity includes such strategies as developing general screening after an apparent suicide cluster; targeted screening; training school and community personnel to recognize verbal and behavioral indicators; presenting general education about youth suicide to staff, students, parents, and the community at large; and forging links to community agencies, such as crisis centers, for appropriate youth referral.

The second level of activity involves school personnel more directly. It includes such strategies as educating staff, students, parents, and community volunteers in the schools about suicide risks and indicators; developing in-school peer support programs; and actively participating in the creation of crisis centers (on-site or off-site) and hotlines.

Programs

Keeping these two levels of activity in mind, the following paragraphs describe basic programs, such as general suicide education, gatekeeper training, screening, peer support programs, crisis centers and hotlines, and means restriction.

General suicide education is an important first step in developing awareness, both of the potential for student suicide and of the need to develop school-based prevention. Such general suicide education provides educators, students, and, hopefully, parents with facts about suicide; alerts them to suicide warning signs; and provides them with information about how to seek help for themselves or others. For students in particular, general education about youth suicide is designed to encourage self-referral for those with suicidal feelings and to increase referrals by peers who recognize suicidal tendencies in someone they know. An effective program of general suicide education incorporates a variety of self-esteem and social-competency development activities.

Gatekeeper training is directed at one or both of two populations. The two populations usually are defined as "school" and "community." The training is designed to help individuals identify students at risk of suicide and to refer such students for help to professional mental health services. School gatekeeper training topics include the signs of youth depression, warning signs for suicide, myths of youth suicide, to whom at-risk youth can be referred, guidelines to follow in making referrals, and the importance of school crisis policies. This type of training increases the confidence and comfort level of school personnel in addressing youth suicide. Such programs also teach staff how to respond in cases of completed or attempted suicide and often include training in school responses to other crises. Annual (renewal) training is recommended for effective intervention (Coy 1995).

Community gatekeeper training is similar in many respects to school training but is directed at such community organizations as service clubs, clergy, police, merchants, recreation facility staff, and governmental groups. Such training is designed to build support for school-based prevention efforts and to help involved community people identify youth at risk of suicide and refer them for help. Training topics include local and national youth suicide statistics, the magnitude of the youth suicide problem, and possible solutions to teen suicide.

One way to initiate the development of a strong community component is to provide a communitywide seminar on "Youth Suicide Prevention" for community service providers, educators, law enforcement, clergy, and parents. A one-day seminar is generally of great interest to the community, stimulates a common dialogue regarding the issue of youth suicide, generates a list of interested and supportive community individuals, and encourages community planning activities (Hicks 1990).

Gatekeepers may find the At-Risk Indicators checklist in Chapter One to be a useful general resource. The Youth Suicide Danger Signs checklist on the next page offers a more targeted list.

Screening for suicide risk usually involves administering some form of risk assessment. Therefore, the question that immediately arises is, What do we screen for? Various experts suggest three areas for consideration: 1) indicators of depression, 2) stressors affecting students, and 3) students' methods for responding to and handling difficult problems. The Depression Alert checklist in Chapter One is an example of one screening tool, which is designed to be used by a teacher or a parent who suspects that a teen may be depressed. Other instruments are available for students to complete that can be useful to school personnel and to the students themselves. Local community health and mental health agencies are the best sources for up-to-date screening instruments and related information. Some local agencies will provide such screening on request and may be amenable to cooperating on programs with the schools.

Peer support programs capitalize on the fact that a student's friends and classmates frequently can discern risk of suicide

YOUTH SUICIDE DANGER SIGNS

Youth who exhibit three or more of the following danger signs should be considered at risk of suicide.

- ☐ Frequent suicidal "talk" as revealed through writing, drawings, or indirect verbal expression.
- ☐ Extreme mood swings (violent or rebellious behavior, sudden cheerfulness, sometimes alternating).
- ☐ Sudden lifestyle changes (activities, manner of dress or expression).
- ☐ Withdrawal or isolation from peers, family, or school activities.
- ☐ Neglect of personal appearance.
- ☐ A history of previous suicide attempt(s).
- ☐ Loss of a special friend (boyfriend, girlfriend, best friend).
- ☐ Giving away prized possessions, putting affairs in order (uncharacteristic cleaning of room or sorting).
- ☐ Decline in school work, failing grades, cheating.
- ☐ Significant change in sleeping habits and energy level (very high or very low).
- ☐ Use of drugs or alcohol.
- ☐ Unexplained absences (from school, work, home).

before that risk becomes apparent to teachers or parents (Davis and Sandoval 1988). A friend often is the first to hear about self-destructive thoughts in a suicidal youth (Ross 1985). This was true in the case of a 17-year-old in Ohio who killed himself. The at-risk youth confided his suicidal thoughts to his friends, but unfortunately they doubted the seriousness of his intentions. Tragically, the friends told no one until it was too late. Ironically, on the night of the young man's suicide, his friends called the family to express their concern for him.

General suicide education is a first step to increasing peer awareness, but the next, more proactive step is to develop formalized peer support. Because a classmate or friend is the most frequent confidant of a suicidal adolescent, teens need to know how to recognize warning signs and when, how, and where to get professional assistance for a troubled peer. Students need to learn that it is essential — sometimes even lifesaving — to take warning signs seriously and, when necessary, to break a confidence (Ryerson 1990).

Peer support programs can be developed and conducted at school or at a community setting, such as a mental health agency, with school cooperation. Such programs are designed to foster positive peer relationships and to develop personal competencies and social skills as a method of preventing suicide among high-risk youth. Peer support programs also include teaching young people how to intervene with peers in order to promote self-esteem, to build skills in handling stress, and to develop support networks for at-risk youth or teens who already have attempted suicide.

Various experts suggest that school officials who want to develop formal peer support groups must 1) use a careful selection process for student participants, 2) develop and conduct a comprehensive suicide education program with a solid peer facilitation component, and 3) provide knowledgeable professional supervision for the students after they have been trained and begin to work with other students (Hart 1989). Peer support groups usually are initiated by interested counselors, psychologists, or social workers already on a school's staff; but the impetus can come from any concerned individual or group. However, the individual implementing or supervising the peer support program should have clinical training and be a licensed counselor, psychologist, or social worker (Lewis and Lewis 1996).

Crisis centers and hotlines provide emergency counseling for suicidal people and usually are staffed by trained volunteers. Many also provide information and referral services in addition to crisis responses. Most crisis centers operate outside the school, usually through a community agency. Some school-based or school-related suicide prevention programs offer a "drop-in" crisis center and referral to traditional mental health services. These programs are designed to encourage self-referral for youth who are experiencing suicidal feelings.

Some at-risk students are unwilling or psychologically unable to engage in face-to-face communication, which makes the telephone hotline a useful tool for suicide prevention. A depressed, suicidal, or questioning teen can call anonymously and seek advice or referral to a community agency. Often, teens at risk simply need to hear another human voice, someone who can respond to them without judging or condemning. Suicidal behavior is often associated with a crisis situation, and the victim can experience ambivalence about living and dying. People have a basic need for interpersonal communication that often will be expressed in a last-minute "cry for help" (Garland and Zigler 1993). The crisis center or the hotline can be the right answer "in the nick of time."

Most school personnel do not become directly involved in the development of crisis centers or hotlines. In any case, developing these programs, training staff, and general oversight should be left to trained mental health professionals.

Means restriction consists of activities designed to restrict access to firearms, drugs, and other common means of suicide. Although means restriction may be critically important in reducing the risk of youth suicide, schools have not placed a major emphasis on this prevention strategy (Centers for Disease Control 1996) — except, of course, to ban such things from school property. But most schools are reluctant to step off the school grounds on this issue. One reason for this reluctance is that means restriction carries implications that are far broader than suicide prevention. At issue are larger concerns that turn on questions of legality and constitutionality, such as restricting access to firearms in the home or making adult purchase of firearms subject to broader supervision by instituting mandatory waiting periods or requiring successful completion of a gun safety course.

Schools can and do restrict student access on school property to firearms and drugs, even to the extent of requiring the mandatory expulsion of any student who brings a weapon onto school property. But beyond the school grounds, the most that educators can do is support stronger measures in the general population. For example, it has been suggested that public awareness campaigns could be undertaken concerning the importance of storing guns and ammunition in separate, locked areas.

Another measure worthy of support from school people would require gun dealers to provide buyers with trigger locks and make the unsafe storage of weapons a felony. Such a law is an alternative to strict gun control legislation, which is more controversial and therefore more difficult to implement (Garland and Zigler 1993).

Additional Recommendations

In addition to the programs discussed above, school officials might consider the following recommendations. These recommendations speak to community relations, program maintenance, and other management issues.

Begin with local support. No suicide prevention effort will succeed that does not have, first, school board support and, second, public approval. School boards set the stage for successful suicide prevention programs by establishing policies that acknowledge the problem and sanction interventions (Hart 1989). Communication beyond the professional community garners program support from parents, community agencies, other community officials, and the general pubic.

Link vital resources. Local support must mature into solid links between the school suicide prevention program and community resources (CDC 1996). In particular, the school program should establish referral procedures that will allow educators to tap the resources of mental health agencies to help manage suicidal crises, treat depressed youth, and collaborate on reintegration when the suicidal teen returns to school after a crisis (Ryerson 1990).

Use multiple prevention strategies. Suicide risk is multidimensional. Therefore, school programs also need to use a variety of

WHEN A STUDENT THREATENS SUICIDE: DO'S AND DON'TS

A young man with a gun turned on himself or a young woman standing on a high ledge is in crisis. What thinking educators do — or fail to do — can make all the difference. Following are some suggestions.

Do —

- Remain calm and stay with the student. Remember, the student is feeling overwhelmed, likely both confused and ambivalent about the suicidal act.
- Get vital information if possible. Ask for the student's name, address, phone number, a parent's work number. Send another student or teacher to get help.
- Clear other students from the scene.
- Assure the student in crisis that he or she is doing the right thing by talking to you. Let the student know that help is on the way and options are available.
- Encourage the student to talk — and listen actively. Acknowledge the student's feelings ("You are really angry," "You must feel humiliated").
- Establish eye contact, speak in a calm voice, and buy time. (Say: "Don't jump. Stand there. Talk to me. I'll listen.")
- Ask the student to agree to a verbal "no suicide" contract. ("No matter what happens, I won't kill myself.")
- Monitor the student's behavior constantly until help arrives. Make mental notes of all the student says; it may be helpful to caregivers later.
- Ensure that the student's parents are informed as soon as possible.

Don't —

- Ignore or minimize a student's threat of suicide.
- Ignore your own intuition about the student's threatening actions.
- Rush the student to talk. Give the student time to think.
- Leave the student alone or allow the student to go anywhere alone, not even to the restroom.
- Lose patience.
- Argue with the student about whether suicide is right or wrong.
- Promise confidentiality. Instead, promise help.

strategies, particularly because no clear indication of effectiveness exists for any single strategy (O'Carroll, Potter, and Mercy 1996). Any good program will begin with basics, such as providing students with opportunities to make decisions and invest themselves in the school, giving praise and recognition, helping students develop self-esteem, and fostering good communication between adults and young people (Page 1996; Kalafat and Elias 1995; Lester 1991). Young people themselves recommend that suicide prevention programs include teaching them skills in communicating, dealing with stress, building self-esteem, and solving problems. They also urge avoiding overuse of the term *suicide*, so that it is not constantly before them (Bolton 1989). Peer counseling rates high on students' list of effective programs, along with posting crisis hotline numbers so that students know where to reach out beyond the school walls.

Incorporate underused strategies. Means restriction is a promising but vastly underused suicide prevention strategy. Peer support groups — particularly related to substance abuse, loneliness, and other at-risk factors — are underused. Many such programs are not specifically targeted for suicide prevention, but they can address issues and problems that often are risk factors for suicide, as well as for running away from home or dropping out of school.

Provide parent education. Parents need to know the suicide warning signs and must be encouraged to restrict teens' access to means for suicide (CDC 1996). Training topics for parents should include: awareness of risks, recognition of warning signs, and basic steps for assisting suicidal youth (Coy 1995). Parents also need to know how to counsel and support the adolescent whose friend may be depressed or suicidal (Ryerson 1990).

Build in program evaluation. Researchers believe that a critical need exists to evaluate suicide prevention efforts, in part to better identify what works and what does not work (Eddy 1989). Examples of areas to evaluate include: the number of suicide victims identified as high-risk before their death, the interventions encountered by a student before suicide, the circumstances surrounding cluster suicides, and so on. Too often a student's death simply marks an end point, but evaluation of the circumstances leading up to that death can help to shape more effective prevention.

I stated earlier that clear evidence of what works and what does not work in adolescent suicide prevention is hard to come by. Certainly long-term research is needed. But a more immediate need is to keep young people safe now. Absence of definitive research should not serve to excuse schools from making the best possible effort to prevent youth suicide. The strategies that are summarized in this chapter represent reasonable, not certain, approaches that schools can use as a starting point to develop their own, individually tailored suicide prevention program.

COMPREHENSIVE SCHOOL-BASED SUICIDE PREVENTION PROGRAM: THE BASIC COMPONENTS

Secondary School Level:
- Faculty Seminars
  - Identification of at-risk youth
  - Assessment strategies
  - Communication skills
  - Referral of suspect youth
- Parent Seminars
  - Identification of at-risk youth
  - Assessment strategies
  - Communication skills
  - Referral of suspect youth
  - Parental denial that their child could be at risk of suicide
  - Parenting the "normal" adolescent
- Student-Peer Education
  - Normal adolescent development
  - Self-evaluation of emotional well-being
  - Identification of a peer at risk
  - Assisting the at-risk peer to help

Middle School Level:
- Faculty Seminars
  - Identification of at-risk youth
  - Assessment strategies

Communication skills
Referral of suspect youth
- Parent Seminars
    Identification of at-risk youth
    Assessment strategies
    Communication skills
    Referral of suspect youth
    Parental denial that their child could be at risk of suicide
    Parenting the "normal" adolescent
- Student-Peer Education
    Normal adolescent development
    Self-evaluation of emotional well-being
    Identification of a peer at risk
    Assisting the at-risk peer to help
    Emphasis on personal interaction and relationships
    Life planning skills curriculum content
    Sexuality
    Stress management
    Daily coping skills
    Self-esteem and personal planning/goals

Elementary School Level:
- Faculty Seminars
    Identifying the child who is depressed
    Links between behavior disorders in children and at-risk
        behavior in adolescents
    Factors arising during childhood that contribute to
        adolescent suicide
    Referral of the child of concern
- Parent Seminars
    Parenting skills
    When to seek help for your child
    Importance of parent-school communication
- Student education
    Death education
    Life planning skills curriculum

Adapted from Barbara Barrett Hicks, *Youth Suicide: A Comprehensive Manual for Prevention and Intervention*, © 1990 by the National Educational Service, 1252 Loesch Road, Bloomington, IN 47404. (812) 336-7700. Used by permission.

TEST YOUR KNOWLEDGE OF HOMOSEXUALITY

Answer true or false to the following statements. The correct answers and brief explanations begin on page 43.

1. Homosexuality is a phase that most children outgrow.
2. It is estimated that nearly 10% of our country's population is predominantly homosexual.
3. Lesbians and gay men usually can be identified by certain mannerisms or physical characteristics.
4. Most homosexuals want to be members of the opposite sex and think of themselves as such.
5. A person develops a homosexual orientation because he or she chooses to do so.
6. Some church denominations have condemned the legal and social discrimination of homosexual men and women.
7. Sexual orientation is established at an early age and there is strong evidence of a biological basis for its development.
8. According to the American Psychiatric Association (APA), homosexuality is an illness.
9. A majority of homosexuals were seduced in adolescence by a person of the same sex, usually several years older.
10. Studies show that the majority of child molesters are gay men.
11. Gay men are at least four times more likely to be victims of criminal violence than are members of the general public.
12. Homosexuals can legally be denied basic civil rights in a number of U.S. states where sodomy laws and anti-homosexual laws exist.
13. Homosexuality is not "natural" because it does not exist in other animal species. Therefore, it can be considered dysfunctional behavior.
14. According to the Kinsey study on sexuality, 60% of all men have had some type of homosexual experience prior to age 16.

15. A gay or lesbian orientation can be the result of a bad sexual experience with a member of the opposite sex.
16. A poor relationship with the same-sex parent may cause a child to develop a homosexual orientation.
17. There is a good chance of changing a person's sexual orientation from homosexual to heterosexual with the proper therapy.
18. In a homosexual relationship one partner usually plays the "husband" (masculine role) and the other plays the "wife" (feminine role).
19. A tenet of the homosexual lifestyle is a desire to avoid parenting and the basic responsibilities and values of family.
20. Gay relationships are usually based on sex and are rarely long-lasting.
21. According to estimates, 10% of the student population of any typical American high school may be homosexual.
22. An estimated 28% of gay and lesbian adolescents drop out of school rather than endure verbal and physical abuse.
23. Most teenagers who contract the AIDS virus are homosexual males.
24. Estimates show that homosexuality is more prevalent among teens in urban areas than in rural areas.
25. Gay and lesbian youth account for approximately one-third of all teen suicides and are two to three times more likely to attempt suicide than their straight peers.
26. An estimated 26% of young gays and lesbians are forced to leave home because of family conflict over their sexual orientation.
27. In England the legal age of consent for men depends on their sexual orientation.
28. Same-sex marriages are legally recognized in Denmark.
29. It is estimated that some 1.5 million homosexuals were exterminated by the Nazis during World War II.
30. There is very little information available to suggest that homosexual persons may have made significant historical contributions to society.

ANSWERS TO
TEST YOUR KNOWLEDGE OF HOMOSEXUALITY

1. *False*. To confuse homosexual orientation with a phase is to deprive the adolescent of the opportunity to achieve a positive sense of self. All adolescents go through phases. Gay and lesbian adolescents are no exception (Raider and Steele 1991).
2. *True*. This finding from the famous Kinsey study (Pomeroy 1972) has been challenged by some other surveys but is still widely supported by most researchers.
3. *False*. The vast majority of gay men and lesbians are not identifiable by looks or mannerisms (Uribe et al. 1993). Although they tend to be somewhat invisible, you probably know more gay and lesbian people than you think.
4. *False*. Homosexuality should not be confused with transvestitism (when a person gets psychological gratification from dressing or assuming the mannerisms of the opposite sex) or transsexuality (when a person strongly desires to assume the physical characteristics and gender role of the opposite sex). Most openly gay persons are comfortable with their gender identity (Obear 1985).
5. *False*. It is well documented that sexual orientation is formed before adolescence, and there is strong evidence of a biological basis for its development (Bell, Weinberg, and Hammersmith 1981; Money 1980). While researchers disagree on the specific "causes" of homosexuality, most agree that some type of predisposition or genetic relationship is involved.
6. *True*. A number of mainstream denominations are currently struggling with traditional church views of homosexuality. Biblical scholar John Boswell (1980) argues that the word "homosexual," as we know it, does not appear in any of the Bible's original texts and that nothing in the ancient Biblical scriptures would have precluded homosexual relations among early Christians.

7. *True*. See answer #5.
8. *False*. The American Psychiatric Association (1974) depathologized homosexuality as a mental illness in 1973 and removed it from the DSM-III-R. The American Psychological Association and the American Counseling Association have adopted similar views.
9. *False*. This is a common misconception, but there is no empirical evidence to support the idea that homosexuality is the result of any type of sexual abuse (Raider and Steele 1991).
10. *False*. According to statistics, more than 90% of child molestation is committed by heterosexual men. There is no correlation between sexual abuse and homosexuality (Star 1979). Homosexuality should not be confused with pedophilia (adult sexual desire directed toward a child) (Boswell 1980).
11. *True*. This crime is known as "gay bashing" and often occurs randomly and without provocation. "Gay bashing" has been on the rise since 1983, possibly as a result of the AIDS crisis (National Gay and Lesbian Task Force 1984).
12. *True*. Only six states have gay/lesbian civil rights laws. Twenty-four states, mostly in the South and Southwest, still retain sodomy laws, making consensual sex between adult homosexuals illegal (Uribe et al. 1993).
13. *False*. Another finding of the Kinsey study is that homosexuality occurs as often in other species as it does in humans. It is a "natural" phenomenon that has been evident in all cultures throughout history (Pomeroy 1972).
14. *True*. Homosexual experimentation in childhood is common and a natural part of exploring one's sexuality. Such experimentation does not necessarily mean that a person will be homosexual as an adult (Uribe et al. 1993).
15. *False*. This is another common misconception. There is no empirical evidence to support the idea that a person becomes homosexual as the result of a poor heterosexual experience, or that a homosexual person can become heterosexual by having a satisfying heterosexual experience (Obear 1985).

16. *False*. The revelation of a child's homosexuality often triggers feelings of guilt and blame for parents. This is unfair, unwarranted, and unsubstantiated by any scientific research (Raider and Steele 1991; Uribe et al. 1993).
17. *False*. Parents may seek a heterosexual conversion for their homosexual child, but the APA has denounced this practice as unscientific, unjustified, unethical, and emotionally scarring (Coleman 1978; Gonsiorek 1988).
18. *False*. This is another common misconception. Most healthy gay and lesbian relationships, like healthy heterosexual relationships, are based on equality and mutual respect. There are no specific "masculine" or "feminine" roles (Obear 1985).
19. *False*. Homosexual people are both products and members of families and cherish these values in the same way that heterosexual people do (Raider and Steele 1991).
20. *False*. The various aspects of homosexual relationships are basically the same as those of heterosexual relationships. Sex is only one of these aspects. Some relationships are healthy and last a lifetime; others do not (Lipkin 1990).
21. *True*. Refer to #1. Percentages of adult homosexuals tend to be higher in larger cities and metropolitan areas. However, because most minor children live with their parents, experts say that homosexual youth undoubtedly exist in every American high school, even though they may be "closeted" and virtually invisible (Uribe et al. 1993).
22. *True*. According to a 1989 study by the U.S. Department of Health and Human Services, the abuse included defacing lockers, sending or leaving notes, taunting, and even beating students. A similar study by the National Gay and Lesbian Task Force (1989) found that 45% of gay men and 20% of lesbians had experienced some type of verbal or physical assault in high school.
23. *False*. According to the U.S. Department of Health and Human Services (1991), risk for AIDS through heterosexual contact is greater among adolescents (especially girls) than among adults. Twenty-six percent of adolescent males who

carry the AIDS virus have been infected through homosexual contact, as compared to 66% in the adult population. Adolescent females account for twice as many reported cases of HIV infection as adult females.

24. *False.* See answer #21.

25. *True.* According to the U.S. Department of Health and Human Services (Feinlieb 1989), the anguish suffered by gay and lesbian youth makes them particularly at risk for suicide.

26. *True.* As a result, a significant number of gay teens find themselves living on the streets, engaging in acts of prostitution to survive, and becoming particularly at risk for sexually transmitted diseases and drug and alcohol abuse (Gibson 1989).

27. *True.* In England the legal age of consent for gay men was recently lowered from 21 to 18. For heterosexuals and lesbians, the age of consent is 16. The history of England's intolerant attitude toward male homosexuality is portrayed in *Maurice*, a novel by E.M. Forster.

28. *True.* Denmark is the only country in the world where same-sex marriages are legally recognized (Boswell 1980).

29. *True.* The mass extermination was part of Hitler's mission to create a "superior race." While Jews were required to wear a Star of David on their clothing for identification purposes, homosexuals were required to wear a pink triangle (Uribe et al. 1993).

30. *False.* Many significant historical figures — including Michelangelo, Tchaikovsky, James Baldwin, Emily Dickinson, Gertrude Stein, Walt Whitman, Tennessee Williams, Dag Hammarskjöld, and Martina Navratilova — have been homosexual, though this information is rarely shared in schools, denying gay and lesbian adolescents access to positive gay and lesbian role models (Raider and Steele 1991; Uribe et al. 1993).

Adapted from Matthew Armstrong, "Creating a Positive Educational Environment for Gay and Lesbian Adolescents: Guidelines and Resources for Staff Development, Curriculum Integration, and School-Based Counseling Services," Master's Practicum Project, Heidelberg College, 1994.

Chapter Four

INCLUSIVE PROGRAMMING FOR GAY YOUTH

In the Introduction to this handbook I noted that gay youth often are invisible, certainly in the school setting in general, but also in suicide prevention efforts. Unfortunately, gay teens are vastly overrepresented in the statistics on attempted and completed suicides. For that reason it is important to take up inclusive programming for gay youth in some detail.

The wall of silence that surrounds many gay youth makes it difficult for schools to provide intervention services, whether for harassment in the hallways or for feelings of depression and suicidal ideation. Many gay or questioning youth believe that secrecy is essential in order to avoid harassment from other students and, sadly, from their teachers and school administrators as well (Hammelman 1993).

Destigmatizing homosexuality altogether is the real solution, but that is a long-term goal to be pursued in society at large, as well as in the microcosm of the school. Nevertheless, schools can serve to lead the way; and some small steps can be taken without undue trauma. For example, to break through the wall of silence surrounding gay and lesbian issues, one school simply invited its gay students to meet weekly at lunch time on an informal basis. These meetings were spent discussing the problems that students were encountering in the school and served to alert school officials to discrimination and to the gay students' feelings of isolation and alienation (Uribe and Harbeck 1992).

Absent healthy, affirming gay role models, gay youth often lead stressful double lives as they struggle with sexual identity questions. When unanswered questions lead to hopelessness, loneliness, and despair, then suicide may seem to be the only way out (Savin-Williams 1994). And in recent years, because AIDS has been associated in the media often almost exclusively with gay men and lesbians, a new self-destructive behavior in gay youth has begun to be seen: purposely contracting HIV (Snowder 1996).

Keeping Gay Youth Safe

Homophobia (literally the fear of homosexuals and homosexuality) poisons the atmosphere of many schools and makes them unsafe for gay and sexually questioning youth — and even for youngsters whose parents are gay or lesbian. The first steps that any school can take to keep gay youth safe — as much from day-to-day harassment as from other, more dramatic risks that might lead to suicide — include the following strategies for managing and decreasing homophobia (Uribe et al. 1993):

- Provide staff training in sensitivity to sexual orientation issues. The preceding quiz, "Test Your Knowledge of Homosexuality," can make a good starting point for a faculty discussion about homosexuality. Another discussion starter is "Homosexuality in the School: Attitudes and Behaviors" on page 50. (More about this strategy in a moment.)
- Include gay and lesbian issues in the curriculum by discussing these topics whenever appropriate, by using readings on gay issues or by gay authors, and by allowing gay issues to be addressed in papers and presentations. The silence surrounding gay issues has been broken in society. Many television programs feature gay characters, and gay issues appear regularly in newspapers and popular magazines. No legitimate reason exists for excluding discussions of gay issues in school classrooms.

- Develop lessons specifically to reduce homophobia. Discuss how homophobia affects the lives of gay and straight students alike. Teach students to avoid name-calling and enforce antidefamation policies. Do not let anti-gay remarks and jokes pass unchallenged.
- Use inclusive language when talking about students, parents, and others. Heterosexism is the presumption that everyone is (or should be) heterosexual. Heterosexist language excludes gay youth and leads to isolation and alienation. Using non-gender-specific language when discussing relationships and partner choices will be helpful.

Developing Nondiscrimination Policies and Practices

None of the preceding strategies is likely to be implemented until school officials take up, preferably formally, the matter of discrimination against homosexual individuals — ideally, including both young people and adults.

School systems should be willing to make a public commitment to ensuring that schools are places free from discrimination, violence, and harassment for *all* students and faculty. That means setting in place policies designed to reduce discrimination in all forms against gay and lesbian students, teachers, and other school employees.

Antidiscrimination policies that are enforced increase the self-esteem and trust of gay youth (Snowder 1996). And these feelings can help to combat isolation, alienation, and the depression that often accompanies the silence on gay issues found in so many schools. But policies without practices are toothless. Teachers, administrators, and counselors need training in sensitivity to gay issues, in crisis intervention, and in violence prevention. In the context of gay issues, educators need to know how to work non-judgmentally with gay youth and how to handle conflicts related to sexual orientation issues. Such work also should address the problems of substance abuse, dropping out, and running away that often characterize gay youth in crisis.

HOMOSEXUALITY IN THE SCHOOL: ATTITUDES AND BEHAVIORS

To deal effectively with gay and lesbian issues that can put students at risk, teachers and administrators may need to begin by examining their own attitudes and behaviors. The following yes/no questions may be useful as discussion starters.

Classroom Interactions

1. Teachers who regard homosexuality in a negative way should be able to request a homosexual student to enroll in another class.
2. I would be willing to discuss homosexuality in the classroom and would integrate into my lessons, when appropriate, factual information about gays and lesbians who made significant contributions to society.
3. It would be difficult for me to deal fairly with an openly gay student.

Counseling

4. Providing a homosexual high school student with supportive materials is appropriate for a teacher or counselor.
5. I would feel comfortable if a student talked to me about his or her sexual orientation.

Student Harassment

6. I would discipline a student for harassing another student suspected of being homosexual.

Remafedi (1994) suggests the following goals for staff inservice programs on gay and lesbian issues. Inservice training should be designed to help teachers and administrators:

- Learn about the special needs of gay students;
- Learn about the health problems of gay youth, such as their high risk for suicide;
- Gather and examine resource materials for responding to the needs of gay students;
- Learn to relate antigay discrimination to other forms of prejudice;

7. I would openly disagree with a faculty member who made a disparaging comment about a suspected homosexual student.
8. I would discipline a student for making derogatory remarks or jokes about homosexuals, in general.

Homosexual Teachers

9. I would feel uncomfortable if my school hired an openly gay or lesbian teacher.
10. Homosexual persons should not be allowed to teach in the public schools.
11. Adolescents who are taught by homosexual teachers will be strongly influenced to become homosexual.

Human Rights

12. Teachers and school counselors, regardless of their own personal stance, have a responsibility to work in school to educate students and lessen prejudicial attitudes about homosexuality in our society.
13. I would be willing to work in my school and community to alleviate discrimination against gays and lesbians.

Adapted from Matthew Armstrong, "Creating a Positive Educational Environment for Gay and Lesbian Adolescents: Guidelines and Resources for Staff Development, Curriculum Integration, and School-Based Counseling Services," Master's Practicum Project, Heidelberg College, 1994.

- Discuss existing negative attitudes toward gay people and how to change them; and
- Learn how to create a safe environment so that gay and lesbian staff members, as well as students, can be open about their sexual orientation.

One way that some inservice presenters have found useful for stimulating heterosexual educators to think about homosexuality is to turn cliché questions upside down by substituting the word, "heterosexuality," for "homosexuality," as shown in the "Heterosexual Questionnaire" on the next page.

HETEROSEXUAL QUESTIONNAIRE

1. What do you think caused your heterosexuality?

2. When and how did you first decide that you were heterosexual?

3. Is it possible that your heterosexuality is just a phase that you may outgrow?

4. Is it possible that you could be changed by a healthy gay relationship?

5. Is it possible that your heterosexuality was caused by a bad relationship with a member of the same sex, or a fear of the same sex?

6. Have you disclosed your heterosexual tendencies to anyone? Wouldn't it be more appropriate to keep these feelings to yourself?

7. Why do so many heterosexuals seem compelled to seduce others into the heterosexual lifestyle?

8. Why do heterosexuals place so much emphasis on sex?

9. Statistics suggest that a majority of child molesters are heterosexual. Do you feel it is safe to expose children to heterosexual teachers?

10. Considering the menace of overpopulation, how would the human race survive if everyone were heterosexual?

11. How can you become a whole person if you limit yourself exclusively to heterosexuality and fail to develop your homosexual potential?

12. A lot of heterosexuals seem to be very unhappy. Would you consider some type of therapy to help you change?

Adapted from Matthew Armstrong, "Creating a Positive Educational Environment for Gay and Lesbian Adolescents: Guidelines and Resources for Staff Development, Curriculum Integration, and School-Based Counseling Services," Master's Practicum Project, Heidelberg College, 1994.

Yet another way of helping educators delve into the issues faced by gay and lesbian students is to read and discuss case scenarios, such as the five that follow (suggested in Armstrong 1994). The first two are designed for counselors:

Lisa

Lisa is a junior. She is a bright, intelligent girl and, academically, is ranked first in her class. She also is popular, attractive, and very involved in school activities. For several weeks you have been hearing rumors that Lisa has been having a lesbian relationship with another student. The rumors have spread to the teachers' lounge, and teachers are concerned because they are beginning to observe negative behaviors displayed toward Lisa in their classrooms. Lisa shows up at your office door at lunch time. You say, "Hi, Lisa. What can I do for you?" Lisa responds by bursting into tears. How do you handle the situation?

Matt

Matt is a sophomore. He is an athlete, a football star, and physically is well-developed for his age. He has a reputation for being something of a "bully" but is generally popular with his classmates. He is an average student and is not highly motivated in the classroom. The words "faggot" and "queer" seem to be his favorite expletives. Matt has been referred to your office by the principal after a phone call from a parent complaining that her son has been harassed both physically and verbally by several "jocks" for weeks. The final straw came when her son, who was getting a drink at the water fountain, was grabbed from behind in the genital area by Matt. How do you proceed?

The following three scenarios are designed for teachers. In the first scenario, Chris can be either male or female, depending on the teacher who is responding to the problem.

Chris

Chris is a 16-year-old junior. You are a single teacher of the same sex as Chris. Chris is a bit of a loner, an average student whose home life is less than ideal. He seems to be making a real effort to do well in your class, and you have tried to give some special attention and positive feedback in the hope that it will help him build a more positive self-image.

One evening Chris shows up at your front door, saying that he really needs to talk to someone. Eventually Chris reveals feelings that he might be gay. When you are supportive and nonjudgmental, the flood gates open. Chris reveals that he has been having intimate homosexual encounters with another student who also is in one of your classes. Now Chris is distraught over the break-up of this relationship and has no one with whom to talk about it. Chris becomes quite emotional and begs you not to tell anyone, especially his parents, who he is sure will throw him out if they discover this secret.

In the weeks to come Chris continues to show up at your home unannounced. Other teachers begin to question what is going on. You are reluctant to break Chris' confidence because of the homophobic attitudes of the school and community, but you fear your own credibility and career may be in jeopardy. You also are concerned that Chris may be developing an infatuation for you. What do you do?

Jeremy

Jeremy is a freshman. He displays a number of stereotypically effeminate characteristics, and occasionally you have heard the words "fag" and "queer" uttered by some students just before Jeremy comes into your classroom. Up to this point, however, you have felt that it was better to say nothing than to draw more attention to the issue.

Today's lesson is about AIDS. You begin a discussion of some of the facts from the students' previous evening's reading assignment. After asking, "Who can tell us what causes AIDS?" you wait for several seconds for a student to raise his or her hand. Into the silence a student calls out, "Why don't you ask the faggot? He should know." Several members of the class begin laughing, and it is obvious that the response is intended to indicate Jeremy. What do you do?

Cindy

Cindy is an 18-year-old-senior and a player on the girl's basketball team. You are Cindy's English teacher. Cindy has been stopping by your room after school recently and has made a number of derogatory comments about her female basketball coach and the coach's frustration with this year's team. She says the coach is yelling at her too much, that she hates basketball this year, and that no one is happy with how things have been going. The coach is very popular in the community, well-liked, and respected.

In a recent English assignment Cindy wrote a story about a high school athlete who was being sexually harassed by her female coach. You suspect that this may be the key to Cindy's frustration with basketball and, possibly, a cry for help. What do you do?

There is no single correct response to these case scenarios, but teachers, counselors, and administrators will find them thought-provoking as starting points for serious discussions of gay and lesbian issues.

Information and Access

Yet another way that schools can reduce the silence on gay and lesbian issues is to provide information and access to information, assistance, and other resources for gay and sexually questioning students.

Part of this access to information goes back to the strategy of inclusive curricula. Students need to hear and participate in discussions of gay issues, often simply by addressing the issues raised on television or in the local newspaper. Print resources on gay issues need to be available in the school library and classroom book collections (Fischer 1995).

Perhaps as important as information on gay issues is the presence (and knowledge of) gay writers of both fiction and nonfiction. The sensibilities of any writer are formed by many influences: race, philosophy, personal experience, ethnicity, language, heritage, and so on. Not least among these influences — but often unacknowledged — is sexual orientation. If teachers discuss how Langston Hughes' writing was influenced by his race, then it is no great stretch to consider how Virginia Woolf's or Walt Whitman's writing might have been influenced by their homosexuality. Breaking the silence on sexuality issues can be affirming for gay youth, because the worth of such authors is validated.

While providing information at school — whether in the classroom, the library, or the counseling office — is important, schools also can offer all students information about resources outside the school. This may consist of posting the names and addresses of local health and human services agencies, providing pamphlets from community groups, and displaying telephone numbers for gay youth information services, health services (such as AIDS hotlines), and suicide emergency hotlines. A number of these types of information are included in the Resources section of this handbook. Especially useful are hotlines staffed by other adolescents trained in peer support (Proctor and Groze 1994).

If these recommendations are used in the schools, they will help to make candid and open discussions more comfortable for educators and students and information about sexual issues more accessible. Students who once struggled in silence, alone and isolated, will be able to find accurate information, sympathetic understanding, and simple acceptance from educators they trust and respect. Changing public opinion is a slow process, but sensitive educators can help gay students learn to accept themselves for who and what they are: human beings completely deserving of the universal human rights of safety, fairness, and justice in the schools. If this can happen, then schools will have taken solid steps toward reducing the risk of suicide for gay youth.

Chapter Five

AFTERMATH OF A YOUTH SUICIDE

For most of this book I have concentrated on preventing adolescent suicide. However, sometimes even the most vigorous prevention efforts fail, and a young person dies. This chapter and the next are concerned with what school people can or should do in this eventuality.

A teenager's suicide is an overwhelming event in the life of a school, but school must continue. In fact, the organized routine of the school schedule provides a secure setting in which those close to the student can work through the bereavement and recovery process. All students need a supportive environment in which to express their grief and to work through their feelings. Teachers and other staff, if properly trained, can be sources of sound information and helpful reassurance, even when they themselves may be feeling a deep personal loss and a sense of failure.

A suicide, like a train wreck, leaves survivors who must deal with complex emotions. One of the most common is a feeling of abandonment. "Now I'm alone. What will I do?" is a natural reaction. The same is true for a sense of rejection. In rejecting life, the youth who takes his own life also rejects the significant others in his life. As one survivor put it: "He could not have loved me; he did not think I was worth living for."

It takes a great deal of effort to come to terms with the fact that young people who kill themselves may be attempting to escape from emotional pain that is quite disconnected from those around them who care deeply.

Survivor Guilt and Social Stigma

Another common feeling among survivors is self-blame, sometimes called "survivor guilt." Parents and peers may blame themselves for not seeing the signs of the impending suicide or for not meeting the needs of the student at risk. Survivors may question what they did to add to the student's stress or wonder why they did not foresee and stop the act. This sense of responsibility was aptly expressed by one teenager in a note to the parents of a classmate who had taken his own life:

> To send mere condolences is not enough. To say only, "I'm sorry," is short and sour, but to say that I have once felt the grief that you all feel now would be more exact. Like your lost son or brother, I know what it is to feel alone and misplaced. If only I had known that we shared that common barrier, I would have reached out, but I failed. Over the years I have realized that aloneness cannot be cured through isolation, and I feel partially responsible because I never let Dick know. The shadow of aloneness consumed Mr. D.J. Now someone else has to play his music. We closed our hands and tuned out his lyrics.

Some young people also fear that others will blame them for the student's death, perhaps because they had rejected the student or had an argument with the student shortly before the suicide. Even after 23 years, one young woman I met would not speak of her father's suicide, which occurred when she was only three years old, because she feared, however irrationally, that people would blame her for his death.

Young people who "survive" the suicide of a close friend or sibling also may worry that they themselves might follow the deceased's self-destructive act. Those closely identified with the suicide victim may begin to see the act of killing oneself as an appropriate resolution to life's problems. Suicide becomes no longer an abstract concept. The taboo has been broken. And suicide gains a kind of validation because it was the path chosen by someone close.

One "survivor," whose daughter took her life, wrestled with suicide issues for 20 years until, in the end, she also took her own life. In outward appearance this individual seemed to be functioning well. She even was active in the community's suicide support group. But she left behind a note that said, "Forgive me; I can no longer bear the pain."

Survivor guilt also can translate into social isolation. Suicide, a taboo act, carries a stigma that can isolate those close to the suicide victim. Not only do "survivors" blame themselves, but they also are subtly tagged with blame by others. Members of the community and the deceased student's peer group may turn away from the victim's close friends and relatives. Avoidance and silence can deepen the sense of loss.

After the suicide of a 17-year-old, his teenage sister said, "Many of my friends and teachers never mentioned my brother's death. I lost a lot of friends at school and always felt so lonely." The older brother of this same suicide victim also commented:

> When I ask my friends how their families are doing, I can almost see an invisible curtain fall between us. Sometimes they don't answer, because then they would be expected to ask about my family. And they don't want to discuss my brother's suicide or the pain of my family.

Parents and peers of gay youth who kill themselves suffer a double dose of shock and grief. And the stigma of suicide may be further strengthened by the societal stigma of homosexuality. Guilt is the most common emotion felt by parents when they learn that their son or daughter is gay (Johnson 1996). Because homosexuality is so often regarded as "unnatural" or "sinful," parents often anguish over what they might have done wrong to cause their child to "turn gay." One parent said that she felt as though she had the word, "FAILURE," written across her forehead.

When a gay youth completes suicide, the kaleidoscope of emotions are compounded for the surviving family, especially if the youth's sexual orientation has been a point of contention. One mother blamed herself and her strong religious beliefs for the suicide of her gay son. She felt responsible for the suicide because, for religious reasons, she had constantly rejected her son's sexual orientation (Aarons 1995). Peers also may be overwhelmed by feelings of guilt — for "making the young person gay," for not accepting the young person's sexual orientation, for not seeing the young person's pain, for not preventing the act of suicide.

Bereavement and Recovery

Often it is said that children have a "natural resilience to emotional pain," but most modern authorities now take the opposite view. One of the destructive, silent myths about children and suicide holds that children do not grieve as deeply as adults do. The myth posits that children may be sad and hurt, but they never experience the anguish and gut-wrenching sorrow of profound grief. In fact, quite the opposite is more often the case. Children grieve deeply but, as in other aspects of emotional life, they may show their grief in ways that are different from adult grief.

The bereavement and recovery process includes five stages, or phases: denial, guilt, anger, acceptance, and resolution (Hewett 1980). These different grief phases or stages do not occur automatically. Not every person will move directly from one to another. By becoming familiar with the characteristics of these five stages, educators can help themselves and their students to better understand their feelings when a student completes suicide.

Denial. On first hearing of a student suicide, the common response is denial. "It can't be true. He was cleaning the gun, and it just went off." Questions and contradictions quickly follow. "It must have been an accident. She wouldn't really do that." "Why did it happen? He couldn't have been serious." "Is there some chance that he is still alive, that the shot wasn't fatal?"

Following a suicide, survivors frequently use denial to mask feelings. And denial is not all bad, because it is one way of holding at arm's length the specter of pain and suffering to come until the mind and heart are more prepared to accept the tragedy (Hewett 1980). In a study of families in which an adolescent completed suicide, denial was manifested in the form of hostility toward the medical examiner and toward anyone who called the death a "suicide." In part, this hostility also reflects the stigma that is associated with suicide.

Of course, there are some realities associated with suicide that reinforce the societal taboo. Some insurance policies, for example, include a "suicide clause" that reduces or eliminates benefits. Some religions deny traditional burial rites to those who die by their own hand. Access to certain religious burial grounds are denied to the suicide victim.

The denial stage may continue through the funeral and burial rites and memorial services. Peers and family go through the motions in a state of shock. Often their faces appear expressionless, and they look to others for behavior to model.

Some students seem to get stuck in the denial stage, refusing for years to discuss the suicide. When a 13-year-old's brother took his own life, the youngster had entered college before he ever again spoke his brother's name. Then he began to write about his brother's suicide in papers for his classes.

Teachers also go through denial when a student they know completes suicide. But they often mask their deeper feelings by dealing with the immediate. One teacher asked, "What do I do with the empty chair where the student sat? Do I remove the desk before the other students come in? Should I mention the student's death?" In fact, the presence of an empty desk or chair may be a way to allow the teacher and the students to express their feelings of loss, to begin the grieving process.

Guilt. Feelings of guilt mark a significant difference between those who experience the death from accident or illness of someone close to them and those whose friend, child, or sibling completes suicide. When suicide is the cause of death, feelings of guilt tend to be far more intense. Suicide is seen as a far more "preventable" death, if only. . . if only (Berman and Jobes 1995).

Feelings of guilt may be further heightened if the young person gave clear signals of intent that were ignored or, worse, disparaged or not taken seriously. How does the educator respond? What words — what self-talk — can avail? In the end, perhaps the best advice is to remember, and to help students remember, that suicide is an act completed in solitude. Only one person is truly responsible: the person who dies (Hewett 1980).

Anger. Past denial, past guilt, there often follows anger. A sibling or classmate may be angry at being left behind, left alone. Or the anger may arise from a sense of the pain to which friends and family have been put by the sudden death and the stigma attached to it.

Some young people will want to lash out in anger. But the suicide victim is beyond their wrath, and so it may turn inward. They may themselves become destructive or self-destructive.

It is important for educators to recognize student anger following the death of a peer, but it also is important for them to recognize the anger within themselves. Anger can be a positive motivator as well as a destructive one. Anger can prompt action. Anger over a death by cancer may prompt one to contribute to scientific research for cancer cures; anger over a death in an automobile accident may prompt one to lobby for stronger safety laws. So, too, can anger over a death by suicide prompt one to redirect energy toward life-affirming activities and suicide prevention work.

One teacher I know has carried on a tradition for 17 years of conducting an annual writing contest in memory of a student who completed suicide. The deceased student's family contributes award money to encourage the development of creative writing skills and so also keeps alive the memory of their lost child.

Acceptance. Student acceptance of the reality and the finality of a suicide may come in a week or a month or a year, but it comes eventually. The victim is gone and will not return. The finality of death is accepted. This is a difficult time for adolescent survivors, but acceptance is a critical step in their recovery.

Educators assist students in coming to terms with a peer's death by being open to discussion, understanding as the students go through the various stages of grieving, and accepting and affirming. To reach the stage of acceptance, students must come to understand that, while someone who once was in their lives

---

DEALING WITH GRIEF

It must not be overlooked that as educators help students deal with feelings of grief, they also will be grieving. These suggestions are for teachers and administrators:

- You may be overwhelmed by the intensity of your feelings. Know that such intense feelings are normal and common.
- You may feel angry at the person who ended his life or at someone close to that person. You may be angry at the world in general. Such anger is common.
- You may feel guilty for what you think you did or did not do. You are not to blame.
- You may feel hopeless and depressed. These feelings are common and in time will pass.
- Remember, you are a person of worth, even though you may not think so at the time.
- Express your feelings to others. Denying or hiding your feelings may lead to depression. If necessary, express your feelings through creative activity.
- Learn about the grief process so that you know what to expect and can explain it to others.
- Call on your personal faith to help you through this emotional time. Allow your friends to comfort you.
- Be part of a support system that includes colleagues and others outside of school. The trauma of a student suicide does not go away at the end of the school day.
- Do not be afraid to use professional help as part of your support system.

---

found self-destruction to be an answer to life's problems, they have other, more affirming options. They can exercise control over their own lives, even in the face of seemingly insurmountable adversity.

Resolution. The final stage is one of "moving on." This is not to say that the dead are forgotten or diminished in value. Sorrowful moments will come and go inevitably. But they do not hang on so oppressively. Life — and living — goes on.

In this chapter I have concentrated on the emotional aftermath of a youth suicide. One cannot separate the emotional from the practical, of course. But some tightness of focus may be useful.

In the next chapter I move from this more emotional focus to the practical question: How should educators "manage" the crisis of suicide? I stated at the beginning of this chapter that a suicide is an overwhelming event in the life of a school, but school must continue. How educators can ensure that school continues in a healthy and affirming way is what I will take up next.

Chapter Six

MANAGING THE CRISIS OF SUICIDE

Suicide, like any crisis at school, raises emotions that can run out of control. Schools should be places of safety and security. When a suicide occurs, safety and security are threatened. School officials must be responsive to the emotional needs of students and, in many cases, of parents as well.

Crises can be managed with information and planning. My goal in this chapter is to describe the components of an effective suicide crisis plan and how that plan can be implemented by a school crisis team.

Building a Crisis Team

An effective crisis team can implement prevention strategies as well as respond after a suicide has occurred. But prevention really is everybody's business. Crisis management is best accomplished by a leadership team that can take responsibility for helping other faculty members and students deal with the aftermath of a suicide. (Some crisis teams also are structured to respond to all types of crises, such as accidental deaths, tornadoes, earthquakes, and bomb threats.)

A typical, building-level crisis team should include the principal, selected teachers, a guidance counselor, a school nurse, a secretary, and a custodian. This team should be trained in grief management and human relations. Their responsibilities can be divided into two categories: proactive and reactive. Proactive responsibilities include:

- Developing a protocol for dealing with a crisis.
- Planning and implementing staff inservice training on adolescent suicide, prevention, and responses.
- Cataloguing community resources and developing liaison relationships with outside agencies.
- Identifying and assisting in the monitoring of students at risk of suicide.

Reactive responsibilities include:

- Providing organizational assistance in the aftermath of a suicide.
- Facilitating communication between levels of authority, with outside resources, and between staff and students.
- Developing follow-up reports and debriefing personnel after a crisis.

This sketch of responsibilities will be clearer as I describe the components of a crisis management plan and how a plan functions in action. Before doing so, however, it would be well to examine how the building-level crisis team is complemented by efforts at the central office level.

At the central office, a similar crisis team might be structured, composed of the superintendent and his cabinet-level administrators, in particular the director of counseling (or pupil personnel services) and the director of school social work. Each building principal (or designee) would serve as the liaison to this central team, and the superintendent's team and the various building principals might sit as an advisory and planning group.

In the main, the responsibilities of the central office crisis team include:

- Supervising and coordinating the efforts of the building-level teams.

- Authorizing expenditures for resource materials, additional staff, and so on.
- Maintaining and disseminating resource and training materials.
- Conducting practice drills, or "mock crises," to sharpen team readiness.
- Evaluating crisis management strategies and prevention procedures.
- Establishing a community support team.

The last item — establishing a community support team — is a further extension of the crisis team concept. Although structured more loosely than the internal crisis teams, this community group should coalesce around the principles of sound crisis management. Members of this community group might include: mental health workers, social workers, clergy, lawyers, judges, and media representatives. The purpose of drawing together these individuals is to coordinate community support that will extend to prevention as well as to assistance during a suicide crisis.

Developing and Implementing a Crisis Plan

An unfortunate example may serve as a warning of what can happen when a school does not have a crisis management plan. The high school in question is a large one, composed of nearly 5,000 students.

One Wednesday the school was hit with the start of a crisis when a popular 10th-grade student killed himself. With no crisis plan to follow, the staff began organizing to deal with the emotional upheaval the following day, on Thursday. As ill-luck would have it, the area was hit by a hurricane later that night, and so on Friday the school was closed.

By Monday, after a weekend of relative calm, school officials assumed the suicide crisis was over. Perhaps, in part, the hurricane and its aftermath were thought to have overridden the suicide crisis. But their assumptions were wrong. That Wednesday another student, the closest friend of the first suicide victim, took his life. The student body erupted in anger and outrage that school officials were unable to contain. A solid crisis management plan might have saved the students, their teachers and administrators, and parents a world of anguish.

Effective crisis management proceeds from a well-developed plan. Following are some of the decisions that must be made in order to develop a workable plan:

- Who will be in charge? When a suicide occurs, who calls the crisis team together? Who directs the work of the team? Who speaks for the school?
- What information should staff have ahead of time? What information should be available — and to whom — during a crisis? How should calls from the media be handled? From parents? Who should school officials notify?
- What support activities should be conducted? For whom? What facilities will be available for support group meeting? For community meetings?

When a plan has been developed that answers these questions, it is good policy to provide staff inservice training in crisis management at the start of each school year. Staff need to know who will be in charge in a crisis situation. They need to know their responsibilities and, as important, what not to do.

Training for secretaries and other office workers is particularly important because they often are on the "front line" when it comes to responding to parents and the media. They need to know what to do, what not to do, and to whom to turn for direction as a crisis unfolds.

One especially useful activity is to hold a "mock crisis," or practice drill. This activity can be conducted on a professional work day when students are not at school. By role playing, staff members can practice doing the kinds of things they may be called on to do in the event of an actual suicide crisis.

When an actual crisis occurs, implementation of the plan must be swift and efficient. Following are typical steps to be taken in implementing a crisis plan. The actual plan and its implementation will depend on the individual circumstances of particular schools and communities. Smaller communities, for example, may not have all of the necessary resources within the community and may have to draw on such resources from larger communities that are nearby.

Step 1. Verify that a suicide has occurred. False information is no basis for action. Contact police, hospital authorities, or the coroner's office to verify that a death has occurred — and ensure that the correct name of the victim is on record.

Step 2. Convene the crisis team. Inform the crisis team of the circumstances of the crisis. Draft a statement for the media. Most schools ask reporters not to disrupt the work of the school by interviewing students or teachers on school property and caution staff not to discuss personal information about the suicide victim.

Step 3. Take action. Implement the crisis plan. Delay feeds rumors and allows negative emotions to build. A generalized response to the crisis often begins with the next step.

Step 4. Inform the student body. A straightforward announcement that a student has died and a simple expression of sympathy for the family is sufficient. If funeral arrangements have been made, that information also can be conveyed. Most schools inform their students with an announcement over the public address system or by delivering a written announcement to be read in each class. Calling a general assembly of the student body for this purpose is not recommended.

Students should be informed that bereavement groups will be established so that those close to the victim will be able to gather and discuss their feelings.

Step 5. Convene a faculty meeting to brief the staff about the suicide crisis. This meeting should reinforce the inservice training provided to the staff at the beginning of the school year. The faculty meeting will serve to remind staff members of their responsibilities and to answer questions.

Step 6. Begin small-group support meetings. Support groups of 15 to 20 students can be convened for students close to the suicide victim. Peer facilitators and counselors should be on hand to conduct these meetings, which may continue to be held on a regular basis for several weeks. However, it is not a good idea to put such groups solely into the hands of a peer facilitator, who may not have the maturity to deal with the emotionally charged issues raised in such groups. An important feature of such groups should be outreach. The question should be asked, "Are there other students who should be with us?"

The dynamics of these small groups deserve comment. It is important for group leaders to maintain the cohesion of the group, at least initially. Some students may want to wander from group to group or to form subgroups without an adult leader. Aimlessness and incidental grouping can be counterproductive. Also, some tension may arise between students who feel varying degrees of closeness to the suicide victim. This tension needs to be dealt with. The understanding must be formed that no one's sense of loss is to be discounted. No one's grief is more or less important than another's.

Step 7. Initiate community resource contacts. Assistance from community agencies is helpful in every case; it is essential should cluster suicides occur, because this phenomenon is beyond the scope of the school.

Step 8. Provide an opportunity for parents to come to school to discuss adolescent suicide, the immediate crisis, and their concerns and questions. It is important as a prevention strategy to urge parents to maintain positive contact with their teenagers at all times immediately following a suicide. Under no circumstances should teens troubled by the crisis be left alone.

Step 9. Provide an appropriate memorial. Some experts argue for returning to "business as usual" as quickly as possible to "deglorify" the suicide by limiting acknowledgment of the death and restricting expressions of grief (Garfinkle et al. 1988). Other experts argue that a memorial service or special commemorative event helps to bring closure to the crisis and promotes healthy feelings in friends and families of the dead youth (Siehl 1990).

I tend to favor the latter response. When school personnel attempt to downplay the significance of the suicide, students and others may view their actions as devaluing the human life that has been lost. And negative repercussions may follow. One principal writes:

> At different times, I was faced with suicides in my school. When the first suicide occurred, students came to me and requested that the school flag be lowered to half-mast in memory of the deceased. I honored their request and received much criticism from the community. Some years later, a second youth suicide occurred. The students again requested me to lower the flag to half-mast. Remembering the prior criticism from the community, this time I did not lower the flag. Had I known then what I know now regarding the aftermath of suicide, and what the repercussions would be in terms of low student morale, I would have stolen back in the night and lowered the flag.

Another consideration that prompts some form of memorial service may be concern for siblings of the suicide victim. The teenage sister of a youth who completed suicide was in the same graduating class as her brother. Twenty years after graduating, she recalled:

> During my last year of high school, four students died during the year: One student died as the result of an injury acquired in a football game; another student died in a car accident; another died of leukemia; and my brother completed suicide. At the graduation ceremonies, the principal mentioned the names of all the deceased students except my brother. I guess she didn't think my brother's name was worth mentioning.

Activities Following the Crisis

I mentioned in Step 6 that support-group meetings may continue for several weeks. In fact, there may be a need for ongoing groups to meet and discuss issues related to grieving even years after the immediate crisis has passed. Such discussion groups may be expanded to include a more generalized focus on grieving over the loss of a loved one under any kind of circumstance.

It should be no surprise that faculty members also can become depressed over the death of a student, and such depression will need to be dealt with in some continuing fashion, either through group discussions or, in some cases, through private counseling.

Experts differ with regard to types of follow-up measure, but there is solid agreement that isolated discussions of suicide with students should be avoided. Far better is placing the discussion of suicide into the broader context of social and emotional issues affecting adolescents. Students should be able to explore their stressors and how they cope with the pressures they feel.

Some schools have used panel discussions that allow a group of students to discuss their feelings about teen issues, including suicide, before their peer group. Successful panels model positive discussion of important issues and can help teachers and group leaders to conduct such discussions more effectively in other settings. Students selected to participate on a panel should be articulate and open, that is, willing to discuss matters such as academic pressures, social pressures, divorce, blended families, and so on. Discussions that touch on moving, adjusting to new school situations, dealing with learning problems, being culturally different, and dealing with a death in the family can be healthy ways of broadening the conversation following the focused crisis of a suicide. This activity also can be expanded to include parents in some discussion forums.

Finally, another follow-up activity that has been used successfully is a student stress program. Students participate in this small-group activity voluntarily, and sessions are treated as confidential. Observers and drop-ins are not permitted. The focus on stress and coping is similar to a support group, but the student stress program is more targeted and has a specific beginning and end. Usually a student stress program is designed to last six weeks, and the group meets weekly at a regular time. The group usually is led by a trained counselor, school social worker, or adolescent psychologist. The structured student stress program can be helpful in moving students to come to terms with the pressures they feel, to put stressors into perspective, and to discover ways to reduce stress. Often a student stress program will specifically focus on pressures felt by students in their particular school or in some class or activity common to all the members of the group.

Chapter Seven

FINAL THOUGHTS

Adolescent suicide is not merely a school problem. It is a problem for the entire community; indeed, for community writ large in our society. But schools can help to address the problem, first, by looking inward and, second, by stimulating the larger community to address the problem more broadly.

For the most part, I have concerned myself in this brief handbook with what schools can do internally to respond to the problem of youth suicide. I have suggested, based on the ideas of experts in the field, a number of preventive measures. I firmly believe that every school must be responsible for instituting an active, comprehensive suicide prevention program. Sadly, every school also must have in place a plan for responding to a youth suicide when (or if) that program falls short.

In this handbook I have laid special emphasis on understanding and addressing the needs of gay youth, because such youth make up an inordinately high percentage of youth suicides. Schools find it difficult to deal with sexual issues, especially when sexual orientation is complicated by issues of religion and morality. But the bottom line is clear. Schools must deal with these issues in order to keep young people safe and to reduce the risk of suicide not just for gay and questioning youth but for all young people.

How do schools effect the second measure? In a very real sense schools have direct access to a significant portion of the community: the parents of the students in their schools. They can reach these individuals by several means, including newsletters, meetings, telephone calls, assemblies, and the like. But this outreach effort need not be limited to parents. It takes little effort to extend communication to the community in general. This extension is important because adolescents, unlike their younger siblings, make their way through the entire community. They shop; they work at part-time jobs; they do volunteer work. Educators who reach out beyond the schoolhouse can affect how parents and other citizens view students and their problems. Schools working with mental health specialists, for example, can make parents and employers of students aware of the pressures that young people feel. One way to do so can be to sponsor or conduct a series of community forums on such topics as drug and alcohol abuse, the pressure to get into college, sexual orientation, and other important matters germane to adolescents.

With regard to gay and questioning youth the schools have a clear stake in helping parents to understand the issues both broadly and, in some cases, with particular reference to their own child. Gibson (1989) suggests that parents need to know and do several things in this regard:

- Parents need to show their gay adolescent acceptance and understanding if the risk of suicide is to be reduced.
- Parents need to be educated about the nature of homosexuality and how sexual orientation develops.
- Parents need to understand the destructiveness of homophobic remarks and behaviors.

These are points of information that also should be known in the community. Gay youth who fear for their safety in the community are also likely to be fearful in school, perhaps in spite of the schools' best efforts to create a safe environment. Therefore, it behooves schools not to limit their efforts to classrooms. In a very real sense the community, too, is a classroom.

Parent education also is a concern in the aftermath of a teen suicide. When a young person dies, parents are shocked and frightened. This is true not only of the parent affected directly but of all parents. Typical questions that parents ask in the aftermath of a youth suicide include: How do I know if my son or daughter is at risk? Should I let my child go to the funeral? Parents need to understand that rarely is a single factor — such as the suicide of a peer — sufficient to put a child at risk. But sharing concerns, talking about feelings, and expressing grief are important post-trauma activities.

Finally, a few words are warranted about the media. While the business of the news media is to inform the public, too often the coverage following a youth suicide is sensational and therefore detrimental. Some evidence exists to suggest that graphic descriptions of the methods employed to complete suicide can influence vulnerable adolescents. Schools can play a role in advising the media of this potential, and responsible media representatives will act with prudence and restraint. In one community, for example, school personnel and mental health professionals expressed their concerns to the executive editor of a large newspaper. As a result, they were invited to give a seminar for local reporters and editors. Subsequent coverage of crisis events was handled with restraint and sensitivity that previously were absent.

Schools also can "manage" a suicide crisis, as I suggested previously, by designating a media contact person. That individual will be responsible for providing the media with reliable information and responses to legitimate questions. By being responsive, providing press releases, and permitting the media to pursue their stories responsibly, schools can reduce inappropriate news coverage that can both deepen the sorrow felt by the grieving and put other adolescents at risk.

In the end, however, it must be said that suicide prevention comes down to individual responsibility. Children must be taught to be responsible for themselves, for managing their feelings and understanding their stresses. Each educator and each parent must take responsibility for this aspect of a young person's education. Only by accepting these personal responsibilities will young people be safe from the risk of suicide.

Resources

Print Resources

Aarons, Leroy. *Prayers for Bobby: A Mother's Coming to Terms with the Suicide of Her Gay Son.* New York: HarperCollins, 1995.

American Psychiatric Association. "Position Statement on Homosexuality and Civil Rights." *American Journal of Psychiatry* 131 (April 1974): 497.

Anderson, John D. "School Climate for Gay and Lesbian Students and Staff Members." *Phi Delta Kappan* 76 (October 1994): 151-54.

Armstrong, Matthew. "Creating a Positive Educational Environment for Gay and Lesbian Adolescents: Guidelines and Resources for Staff Development, Curriculum Integration, and School-Based Counseling Services." Master's Practicum Project, Heidelberg College, 1994. EDRS ED 386613.

Bell, A.P.; Weinberg, M.S.; and Hammersmith, S.K. *Sexual Preference: Its Development in Men and Women.* Bloomington: Indiana University Press, 1981.

Bennett, Roger V. "A Report: Suicide Prevention and Postvention: Perceptions of Counselors, Teachers, and Principals." Paper presented at the American Educational Research Association Annual Meeting, New York, April 1996.

Berman, Alan L., and Jobes, David A. "Suicide Prevention in Adolescents (Age 12-18)." *Suicide and Life-Threatening Behavior* 25 (Spring 1995): 143-53.

Bernhardt, Greg. "Suicide and Mental Illness." *The Ultimate Rejection*, Dayton, Ohio, Suicide Prevention Center newsletter (July 1984): 16-18.

Bolton, I. "Perspectives of Youth." In *Report of the Secretary's Task Force on Youth Suicide, Vol. 4, Prevention and Intervention in Youth Suicide.* DHHS Publication Number (ADM) 89-1623. Washington, D.C.: U.S. Government Printing Office, 1989.

Boswell, J. *Christianity, Social Tolerance, and Homosexuality.* Chicago: University of Chicago Press, 1980.

Brent, D.A.; Perper, J.A.; Goldstein, C.E.; Kolko, D.J.; Allan, M.J.; Allman, C.J.; and Zelenek, J.P. "Risk Factors for Adolescent Suicide: A Comparison: Adolescent Suicide Victims with Suicidal Inpatients." *Archives of General Psychiatry* 45 (1988): 581-88.

Cantor, P.C. "Young People in Crisis: How You Can Help." Paper presented to the National Committee on Youth Suicide Prevention and the American Association of Suicidology, Denver, 1987.

Capuzzi, Dave, and Gross, Douglas. *Youth at Risk*. Alexandria, Va.: American Association for Counseling and Development, 1989.

Centers for Disease Control (CDC). *Youth Suicide Prevention Programs: A Resource Guide*. Washington, D.C.: U.S. Department of Health and Human Services, Public Health Service, National Center for Injury Prevention and Control, 1996.

Cochran, K.S., and Turner, A.L. *Adolescent Suicide and the Role of the School as Seen by Secondary School Principals*. Commerce: Texas State University, 1986. ERIC Document Reproduction Service No. ED 297 4741.

Coleman, E. "Toward a New Model of Treatment of Homosexuality: A Review." *Journal of Homosexuality* 3 (1978): 345-59.

Colorado State Dept. of Education. *Be Aware, Be Prepared: Guidelines for Crises Response: Planning for School/Communities*. Denver, 1990. ERIC Document Reproduction Service No. ED 330 919.

Colt, George Howe. *The Enigma of Suicide*. New York: Summit Books, 1991.

Coy, Doris Rhea. "The Need for a School Suicide Prevention Policy." *NASSP Bulletin* 79 (April 1995): 1-9.

Davis, John M., and Sandoval, Jonathan. "Strategies for the Primary Prevention of Adolescent Suicide." *School Psychology Review* 17, no. 4 (1988): 559-69.

Eddy, D.M. "Estimating the Effectiveness of Interventions." In *Report of the Secretary's Task Force on Youth Suicide, Vol. 4, Prevention and Intervention in Youth Suicide*. DHHS Publication Number (ADM) 89-1623. Washington, D.C.: U.S. Government Printing Office, 1989.

Elkind, David. *All Grown Up and No Place to Go: Teenagers in Crisis*. New York: Addison-Wesley, 1987.

Feinlieb, M.R., ed. *Report of the Secretary's Task Force on Youth Suicide, Vol. 3, Prevention and Intervention in Youth Suicide*. DHHS Publication Number (ADM) 89-1623. Washington, D.C.: U.S. Government Printing Office, 1989.

Fischer, Debra. "Young, Gay . . . and Ignored?" *Orana* 31 (November 1995): 220-32.

Garfinkle, Barry D. "School-Based Prevention Programs." In *Report of the Secretary's Task Force on Youth Suicide, Vol. 4, Prevention and Intervention in Youth Suicide.* DHHS Publication Number ADM 89-1623. Washington, D.C.: U.S. Government Printing Office, 1989.

Garfinkle, Barry D.; Crosby, Emeral; Herberet, Myra R.; Matus, Abraham L.; Pfeifer, Jerilyn K.; and Sheras, Peter L. *Responding to Adolescent Suicide.* Bloomington, Ind.: Phi Delta Kappa Educational Foundation, 1988.

Garland, A.F.; Shaffer, D.; and Whittle, B. "A National Survey of School-Based Adolescent Prevention Programs." *Journal of the American Academy of Child Adolescent Psychiatry* 28 (1989): 931-34.

Garland, A.F., and Zigler, E. "Adolescent Suicide Prevention: Current Research and Social Policy Implications." *American Psychologist* 48, no. 2 (1993): 169-82.

Gibson, P. "Gay and Lesbian Youth Suicide." In *Report of the Secretary's Task Force on Youth Suicide, Vol. 3, Prevention and Intervention in Youth Suicide,* edited by M.R. Feinlieb. DHHS Publication Number (ADM) 89-1623. Washington, D.C.: U.S. Government Printing Office, 1989.

Giffin, Mary. "Cries for Help." *Guideposts* (July 1980): 32-35.

Gonsiorek, J.C. "Mental Health Issues of Gay and Lesbian Adolescents." *Journal of Adolescent Health Care* 9, no. 2 (1988): 114-22.

Grazman, Harriet B. "An Open Letter to School Administrators and Mental Health Professionals About School-Based Suicide Prevention Programs." Paper presented to the American Orthopsychiatric Association, Study Group on Adolescence, Toronto, March 1991.

Hammelman, Tracie L. "Gay and Lesbian Youth: Contributing Factors to Serious Attempts or Considerations of Suicide." *Journal of Gay and Lesbian Psychotherapy* 2, no. 1 (1993): 77-89.

Hart, T.E. *Student Stress and Suicide: How Schools Are Helping.* Eugene: Oregon School Study Council, 1989. ERIC Document Reproduction Service No. ED 303 887.

Herdt, G. "Introduction: Gay and Lesbian Youth, Emergent Identities, and Cultural Scenes at Home and Abroad." *Journal of Homosexuality* 17, nos. 1-2 (1989): 1-42.

Hershberger, Scott L., and D'Augelli, Anthony R. "The Impact of Victimization on the Mental Health and Suicidality of Lesbian, Gay, and Bisexual Youths." *Developmental Psychology* 31, no 1 (1995): 65-74.

Hewett, John. *After Suicide*. Philadelphia : Westminster Press, 1980.

Hicks, Barbara Barrett. *Youth Suicide: A Comprehensive Manual for Prevention and Intervention*. Bloomington, Ind.: National Educational Service, 1990.

Hunter, Joyce. "Violence Against Lesbian and Gay Male Youth." *Journal of Interpersonal Violence* 5 (September 1990): 295-300.

Jennings, L. "Suicide Urges a New Search for Safeguards." *Education Week*, 20 September 1989, pp. 2, 20.

Johnson, Barbara. *I'm So Glad You Told Me What I Didn't Wanna Hear*. Dallas: Word, 1996.

Kalafat, John, and Elias, Maurice J. "Suicide Prevention in an Educational Context: Broad and Narrow Foci." *Suicide and Life-Threatening Behavior* 25 (Spring 1995): 123-33.

Lester, D. "State Initiatives in Addressing Youth Suicide: Evidence for Their Effectiveness." *Social Psychiatry and Psychiatric Epidemiology* 27 (November 1991): 75-77.

Lewis, Max W., and Lewis, Arleen C. "Peer Helping Programs: Helper Role, Supervisor Training, and Suicidal Behavior." *Journal of Counseling and Development* 74 (January/February 1996): 307-13.

Lipkin, A. *A Staff Development Manual for Anti-Homophobia Education in the Secondary Schools*. Cambridge, Mass.: Harvard Graduate School of Education Project, 1990.

Mallet, Eleanor. "Robbie's Story." *Cleveland Plain Dealer*, 6 April 1997, pp. 1A, 12A.

Martin, A. Damien. "Learning to Hide: The Socialization of the Gay Adolescent." *Adolescent Psychiatry* 10 (1982): 52-63.

Maslow, Abraham H. *Motivation and Personality*. 2d ed. New York: Harper & Row, 1970.

McKenry, P.C.; Tishler, C.L.; and Kelley, C. "The Role of Drugs in Adolescent Suicide Attempts." *Suicide and Life-Threatening Behavior* 13 (Fall 1983): 166-175.

Money, J. *Love and Love Sickness: The Science of Sex, Gender Difference. and Pairbonding*. Baltimore: Johns Hopkins University Press, 1980.

National Center for Health Statistics. *Advanced Report of Mortality Statistics, 1994*. Prepared for the American Association of Suicidology by John McIntosh. Washington, D.C., 1996.

National Gay and Lesbian Task Force. *Anti-Gay/Lesbian Victimization: A Study by the NGLTF in Cooperation with Gay and Lesbian Organizations in Eight U.S. Cities*. New York, 1984.

National Gay and Lesbian Task Force. *About Coming Out.* Pamphlet. Washington, D.C., 1989.

Obear, K. *Opening Doors to Understanding and Acceptance: A Facilitator's Guide to Presenting Workshops on Gay and Lesbian Issues.* Washington, D.C.: National Gay and Lesbian Task Force, 1985.

O'Carroll, Patrick W.; Potter, Lloyd B.; and Mercy, James A. *Youth Suicide Prevention Programs: A Resource Guide (Summary).* Washington, D.C.: U.S. Department of Health and Human Services, National Center for Injury Prevention and Control, 30 September 1996.

Page, Randy M. "Youth Suicidal Behavior: Completions, Attempts, and Ideations." *High School Journal* 80 (October/November 1996): 60-65.

Pomeroy, W.B. *Dr. Kinsey and the Institute for Sex Research.* New York: Harper & Row, 1972.

Proctor, Curtis D., and Groze, Victor K. "Risk Factors for Suicide Among Gay, Lesbian, and Bisexual Youths." *Social Work* 39 (September 1994): 504-13.

Raider, M., and Steele, W. *Working with Families in Crisis: School-Based Intervention.* New York: Guilford, 1991.

Range, Jerry. "Class." Dayton, Ohio, *Journal Herald,* 8 February 1986.

Remafedi, Gary, ed. *Death by Denial: Studies of Suicide in Gay and Lesbian Teenagers.* Boston: Alyson, 1994.

Remafedi, Gary; Farrow, James; and Deisher, Robert. "Risk Factors for Attempted Suicide in Gay and Bisexual Youth." *Pediatrics* 87 (June 1991): 869-75.

Rofes, E.E. *"I Thought People Like that Killed Themselves": Lesbians, Gay Men and Suicide.* San Francisco: Grey Fox Press, 1983.

Ross, C.P. "Teaching Children the Facts of Life and Death: Suicide Prevention in the Schools." In *Youth Suicide,* edited by M.L. Peck, N.L. Farberow, and R.E. Litman. New York: Springer, 1985.

Ross, C.P. "School and Suicide: Education for Life and Death." In *Suicide in Adolescence,* edited by R.F.W. Diekstra and F. Hawthon. Dordrecht: Martinus Nyhoff, 1987.

Ryerson, Diane. "Suicide Awareness Education in Schools: The Development of a Core Program and Subsequent Modifications for Special Populations or Institutions." *Death Studies* 14 (1990): 371-90.

Sandoval, Jonathan; London, Melinda D.; and Rey, Toni. "Status of Suicide Prevention in California Schools." *Death Studies* 18 (November 1994): 595-608.

Savin-Williams, Ritch C. "Verbal and Physical Abuse as Stressors in the Lives of Lesbian, Gay Male, and Bisexual Youths: Associations with School Problems, Running Away, Substance Abuse, Prostitution, and Suicide." *Journal of Consulting and Clinical Psychology* 62 (April 1994): 261-69.

Schleis, P., and Hone-McMahan, K. "Growing Up Gay: Gay Teens See Few Allies in School." *Beacon Journal*, Akron, Ohio, 4 and 5 January 1998.

Schneider, Stephen G.; Farberow, Norman L.; and Kruks, Gabriel N. "Suicidal Behavior in Adolescent and Young Adult Gay Men." *Suicide and Life-Threatening Behavior* 19 (Winter 1989): 381-94.

Shaffer, David; Fisher, Prudence; Parides, Michael; Hicks, R.H.; and Gould, Madelyn. "Sexual Orientation in Adolescents Who Commit Suicide." *Suicide and Life-Threatening Behavior* 25, Suppl. (1995): 64-71.

Shaffer, David; Garland, A.; Gould, M.; Fisher, P.; and Trautman, P. (1988). "Preventing Teenage Suicide: A Critical Review." *Journal of the American Academy of Child and Adolescent Psychiatry* 30 (November 1988): 588-96.

Shneidman, E.S. *Definition of Suicide.* New York: John Wiley & Sons, 1985.

Siehl, P.M. "Suicide Postvention: A New Disaster Plan - What a School Should Do when Faced with a Suicide." *School Counselor* 38 (September 1990): 52-57.

Snowder, Frances. "Preventing Gay Teen Suicide." In *Open Lives, Safe Schools*, edited by Donovan R. Walling. Bloomington, Ind.: Phi Delta Kappa Educational Foundation, 1996.

Star, B. "Research Perspectives on the Impact of Sexual Abuse." In *Proceedings of the Fourth National Conference on Child Abuse and Neglect.* Washington, D.C.: U.S. Department of Health, Education, and Welfare, 1979.

Treadway, Leo. "Creating a Safer School Environment for Lesbian and Gay Students." *Journal of School Health* 6 (September 1992): 352-57.

Uribe, Virginia, and Harbeck, Karen M. "Project 10 Addresses Needs of Gay and Lesbian Youth." *Education Digest* 58 (October 1992): 50-54.

Uribe, V., et al. *Project 10 Handbook: Addressing Lesbian and Gay Issues in Our Schools. A Resource Directory for Teachers, Guidance*

Counselors, Parents, and School-Based Adolescent Care Providers.
5th ed. Los Angeles: Friends of Project 10, 1993.
U.S. Department of Health and Human Services. *Preventing HIV Infection Among Youth.* Rockville, Md., 1991.
Wenz, F.V. "Sociological Correlates of Alienation Among Adolescent Suicide Attempts." *Adolescence* 14 (Spring 1979): 19-29.
Werner, E.E. "High Risk Children in Young Adulthood: A Longitudinal Study from Birth to 32 Years." *American Journal of Orthopsychiatry* 59 (January 1989): 72-81.
Wolfle, Jane A. "School Suicide Prevention Programs: Recommendations from Five New Studies of Students, Teachers, Counselors and Principals." Paper presented at the Association of Teacher Educators Annual Conference, Washington, D.C., February 1997.
World Health Organization. *World Health Statistics Annual, 1990.* Geneva, Switzerland, 1991.

Organizations

American Association of Suicidology
2459 Ash Street
Denver, CO 80222
(303) 692-0985
National clearing house on suicide issues.

Bridges Project of American Friends Service Committee
1501 Cherry Street
Philadelphia, PA 19102
(215) 741-7133
Advocates for the establishment of youth-serving organizations.

Gay, Lesbian, and Straight Education Network (GLSEN)
121 West 27th Street, Suite 804
New York, NY 10001
(212) 727-0135
Advocates respect for all students regardless of sexual orientation.

Indiana Youth Group (IYG)
P. O. Box 20716
Indianapolis, IN 46220
(317) 541-8726
Model youth-serving agency with satellite chapters in Indiana.

National Advocacy Coalition on Youth and Sexual Orientation
1025 Vermont Avenue, N.W., Suite 200
Washington, DC 20005
(202) 783-4165
Lobbying and education agency in support of gay youth.

National Coalition for Gay, Lesbian, and Bisexual Youth
P. O. Box 24589
San Jose, CA 95154-4589
(408) 269-6125
Provides referral services on an outreach basis for youth.

National Gay and Lesbian Task Force
2320 17th Street, N.W.
Washington, DC 20009-2702
(202) 332-6483
Policy institute for the elimination of injustice against gay and lesbian people.

National Network of Runaway and Youth Services
1319 F Street, N.W., Suite 401
Washington, DC 20004
(202) 783-7949
Provides technical assistance, training, and HIV/AIDS resources.

PFLAG (Parents, Families, and Friends of Lesbians and Gays)
1101 14th Street, N.W., Suite 1030
Washington, DC 20005
(202) 638-4200
National group; community groups across the United States.

Project 10
7850 Melrose Avenue
Los Angeles CA 90046
(213) 651-5200, ext. 244
Educational information about gay youth for schools.

About the Author

Wanda Y. Johnson is an adjunct assistant professor of educational psychology at Wright State University in Ohio. Previously she taught at Bowling Green State University, and she was an educator in the Dayton Public Schools for 14 years. She holds a Ph.D. in educational leadership from the University of Dayton.

Wanda Johnson has written numerous articles on teen suicide and has been a frequent presenter on this topic for state and national audiences. She also has facilitated support groups for survivors of suicide in Montgomery and Auglaize Counties in Ohio. She and her husband, Richard, live near Dayton, Ohio, and are the parents of four children: Tony, Dick, Robin, and Jerry.